Supporting the Transition from Breastfeeding

by the same author

Supporting Breastfeeding Past the First Six Months and Beyond
A Guide for Professionals and Parents
Emma Pickett
ISBN 978 1 78775 989 3
eISBN 978 1 78775 990 9

of related interest

Breastfeeding Twins and Triplets
A Guide for Professionals and Parents
Kathryn Stagg
ISBN 978 1 83997 049 8
eISBN 978 1 83997 050 4

Supporting Autistic People Through Pregnancy and Childbirth
Hayley Morgan, Emma Durman and Karen Henry
ISBN 978 1 83997 105 1
eISBN 978 1 83997 106 8

Supporting the
Transition
from
Breastfeeding

A Guide to Weaning for Professionals,
Supporters and Parents

Emma Pickett

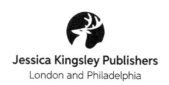

Jessica Kingsley Publishers
London and Philadelphia

First published in Great Britain in 2024 by Jessica Kingsley Publishers
Part of John Murray Press

2

A CIP catalogue record for this title is available from the
British Library and the Library of Congress

ISBN 978 1 83997 785 5
eISBN 978 1 83997 786 2

Printed and bound by CPI Group (UK) Ltd, Croydon, CR0 4YY

Jessica Kingsley Publishers' policy is to use papers that are natural, renewable and recyclable
products and made from wood grown in sustainable forests. The logging and manufacturing
processes are expected to conform to the environmental regulations of the country of origin.

Jessica Kingsley Publishers
Carmelite House
50 Victoria Embankment
London EC4Y 0DZ

www.jkp.com

John Murray Press
Part of Hodder & Stoughton Limited
An Hachette UK Company

To you, if you are struggling with how to balance your own needs with your children's – especially if you are sleep deprived.

Contents

Disclaimers/Notes on Text

This book is written from the perspective of a parent who breastfed and raised children in the UK and supports UK parents as a professional. I acknowledge that I am limited in my understanding by my own experiences, privilege and cultural background. All quotes given by parents and professionals are shared with consent.

The term 'weaning' is used differently in the English language and that can result in some confusion. It comes from the Anglo-Saxon word *wenian*, meaning 'to become accustomed to something different'. It has been used to refer to the introduction of solid food (which is one step in a longer weaning journey). In this book, 'weaning' refers to the end of breastfeeding. 'Starting solid food' will be used to describe when the baby starts to eat complementary foods other than human milk. 'Child-led weaning', or 'self-weaning', refers to when a child takes the lead in stopping breastfeeding. This is distinct from baby-led weaning, which is a method of introducing solid food at six months where the child is not fed by an adult with a spoon but moves directly to self-feeding food which they pick up and manipulate themselves, as part of a family meal.

Lactation support is about centring the families we support and helping them on their journeys at a time when they may often feel isolated. Not all families we support use the term 'breastfeeding' and may prefer 'chest-feeding', 'nursing' or a word individual to their family. Not all parents who feed their children are 'mothers'.

This book's content is for informational purposes only and is not intended to serve as a substitute for the consultation, diagnosis and/

or medical treatment of a qualified physician or healthcare provider. There may be individual cases where a child is dependent on human milk for nutritional reasons and ending breastfeeding needs extra-careful consideration. Stopping breastfeeding can also subject the parent to the risk of health conditions such as mastitis and abscesses, and additional monitoring may be needed.

Chapter 1

Introduction

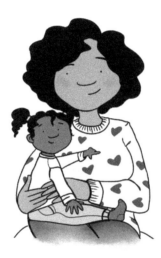

For those of us involved in supporting breastfeeding, whether as a professional or a volunteer, our day-to-day challenge is helping families to get breastfeeding off to a good start. We want a parent to reach their feeding goals and we breathe a sigh of relief when weight gain is good, the pain has eased and the parent and nursling are making breastfeeding work. We can file away a set of notes and move on to the next family. But we may be struggling to support mothers who feel isolated. They may only have had access to overstretched health professionals and may be overcoming a birth which didn't go to plan and had an impact on the entire family. As breastfeeding supporters, we don't often meet the parents who find it all plain sailing. There are enough breastfeeding challenges in the world to fill a career five times over. It is never possible to support everyone who needs our help and, as a profession, we often need to work especially hard to put boundaries in place and practise self-care. As Professor Amy Brown describes in her book examining the experiences of lactation professionals, *The Compassion Code*:

> Working in lactation support can feel like an uphill battle because it is. You are fighting against a system that often undervalues breastfeeding, mothers and new families. Fires have to be put out and problems fixed before you can start at the beginning. (Brown 2022, p.60)

You may work in a hospital and have little interaction with parents at the next stage of their breastfeeding experience. You may volunteer in a support group where nurslings over a specific age aren't ever expected to be brought through your door or are even permitted. However, breastfeeding continues beyond that initial phase and is often out of our sight. It may continue for weeks or years, and when it comes to the end of that experience, our expertise is desperately needed. It is not just our knowledge of lactation and breast health that is valuable but our empathy, our counselling skills and our understanding that breastfeeding, and ending breastfeeding, can bring up complex feelings.

Support to end breastfeeding, particularly after the first year, is lacking and parents are suffering. There are several different problems. Not everyone who works in breastfeeding support does have personal experience of breastfeeding older children (or breastfeeding at all). You may not even realize what the day-to-day parenting of a breastfeeding toddler or pre-schooler looks like. You may not appreciate the central role that breastfeeding can come to have in almost every aspect of parenting: calming, soothing, entertaining, connecting and aiding sleep. Your training probably paid little attention to how breastfeeding ends. Then we have the issue that those who hold the purse strings usually care little about what happens at the end of breastfeeding. What is the motivation for a local community to fund weaning support groups (or ensure it is covered in training) when all the measurable goals are about breastfeeding for six weeks, four months or six months? Whether or not a parent exclusively breast-feeds for six months has a population-level impact on a country's health outcomes, health expenditure and even GDP. Whether parents feel supported to end breastfeeding between 18 months and 5 years is far more wishy-washy. As those who do have more knowledge and experience to offer, we may not be available. Inevitably, we prioritize the *urgent* and important, not the less urgent and important. Usually, the end of breastfeeding does not need to happen right then or even that week (though there are exceptions, as we will discuss later).

There is also an assumption that 'the breastfeeding community' can cover this one. Parents are in Facebook groups, WhatsApp groups and following Instagram accounts. If they have been breastfeeding for more than a few weeks, they have likely found their online family. There are large Facebook groups with tens of thousands of members. We can see images of breastfeeding, and especially feeding older children, being shared widely. Families are swapping their stories, and continuing to breastfeed is being normalized. However, this rich community of breastfeeding advocacy is not always comfortable with finding space for supporting parent-led weaning. In the last few years, so much energy has gone into celebrating the continuation of breast-feeding that I would argue we are in a phase where we haven't learnt how to cherish toddlers and pre-schoolers who breastfeed, alongside giving support to those who desperately want to stop.

Perhaps it's never going to be possible to hold space for both of those things at the same time, but we certainly have some way to go in terms of trying. Posts on social media say things like, 'Every child weans at their own pace' or 'Normalize nursing to natural term. Self-weaning usually happens between two and seven years old.' We can read poems where the poet is a mother talking to her nursling: 'The only view that matters is yours and yours alone...'. We see photo after photo of older children breastfeeding, now that social media companies have largely got over their initial problems with perceiving breastfeeding as nudity. All this is beautiful and special and thank goodness for it. It feels as though finally we have a home for longer-term breastfeeding. But now imagine you are a mother of a two-year-old and you are breastfeeding and are wretchedly miserable and desperate to stop. How does this world look to you now? There seems to be a contradiction between promoting breastfeeding of older children and natural-term breastfeeding while giving space to ending breastfeeding at any age. In most cases, and most contexts, we do not know how to do both simultaneously.

In some cases, parents and even health professionals don't appreciate that ending breastfeeding might bring challenges. They might imagine that bottles replace the breast universally and there is barely a raised eyebrow. They may be bewildered by the notion that, in some families, ending breastfeeding is the most distressing parenting experience to be faced. Some imagine that milk just naturally tapers off and that's when the toddler detaches themself and waves a fond farewell. They believe that the milk goes away first, perhaps as early as under 12 months. Milk production continues as long as there is stimulation. That may not always be the case if there are certain medications involved or if there is a second pregnancy, but even in the cases when the milk does diminish, that does not always dissuade an enthusiastic nursing toddler.

One of the sparks for writing this book was noticing a post on Facebook. A mother was discussing her final breastfeed. It is a clue that the end of breastfeeding is parent-led when someone knows when their final feed is and even has a photo of it. She posted a photo of her first ever breastfeed and her last ever breastfeed side-by-side. In her post, she explained that she had been in tears during her last ever feed but that it was time to stop, and she still felt OK about her decision. What was her motivation for posting? It seemed as though she was looking for recognition and acknowledgement that she had fed her child far longer than most do. She was proud of her achievement and eager to share her feelings with her community. The responses were interesting. There were certainly a few which shared a sense of celebration; what was striking were the ones that did not. Comments were along the lines of, 'This is sad to see. It looks like neither of you was ready,' and, 'She's still so little' (less than 0.5 per cent of UK children are breastfed to a similar age). There was also an 'I'm so glad I was able to practise child-led weaning and *my* child chose when our breastfeeding relationship was to come to an end.' These were comments in a group purportedly supportive of breastfeeding parents. Again, it seemed that natural-term breastfeeding was considered synonymous with child-led weaning and anything 'less' than that was honestly a bit dirty. Even if only one of those comments had been negative, even if only one out of one hundred, that would sting for that mother and any other mother who feels like she needs to take control of the end of her breastfeeding experience. In some of the larger support groups online, a parent will typically introduce the concept of weaning by asking for no shaming or judgement, but they may still receive some from parents who have strong beliefs in the value of older children continuing to receive breastmilk. I have huge sympathy for the admin of these groups who are trying to walk a delicate line.

How can we overcome the challenge of promoting natural-term breastfeeding and empowering parents to end breastfeeding when it is right for them? The answer has to come from highlighting the importance of parental self-care. We pay lip service to it. We share posts of scented candles and yoga positions, and we talk about mindfulness and meditation apps. We make jokes about gin and bottles of red wine opening at the end of the day, but deep down, we often hold the view that the 'perfect' mother never focuses on herself. Our self-care must fit into spaces that are convenient for everyone else in the family. Mothers often ask permission from their partner to have a bath or even read a magazine for a few minutes. When I first started to hold my online weaning support groups, it was striking how mothers who had continued to breastfeed had often continued with 'responsive breastfeeding' from babyhood into toddlerhood and beyond, and never really allowed themselves to find a balance with caring for themselves.

This is particularly true with parents who may have spent limited time among families with children of different ages before and during the pandemic. They had never seen the transition to parenting an older child up close and were now attempting it themselves with little experience. They started considering weaning from breastfeeding still without permitting themselves to do it for themselves. So often, the reasons were 'My toddler needs more sleep' or 'I'd like him to spend more time with his grandparents'. We will discuss later that a starting point is supporting parents to reflect on their motivations for weaning and, crucially, to permit themselves to care about themselves. It is also valuable for their nurslings to see them caring about themselves. We don't expect two- or three-year-olds to have a full understanding that their needs don't always come first, but we have to start somewhere. An early 'homework' at one of my weaning groups was for a parent to do something for themselves in front of their child. That might mean some yoga but not focusing on the toddler. The session would be focused on themself while the toddler watched television or played independently. Too often, a mother would only consider such a thing if a babysitter was involved, or the toddler was asleep. Some of my group members read their own book in the presence of their awake child for the very first time.

When breastfeeding first begins, a child may be entirely dependent on their parent for nutrition if they are exclusively breastfeeding. We perceive that the child has an inalienable right to food and therefore a right to the breast. As psychotherapist Amanda Leon-Joyce describes (2022), we can get stuck in that mindset. She describes how that right lessens as time goes on and we need to continue 'moving with them' as they become more independent and get their nutrition in other ways. Nurslings can begin to experience that right being withheld. Parents need to understand that their child's right to their breast transitions.

When we talk about natural-term breastfeeding, we need to reaffirm that there are two partners involved in the process. Not the parent who breastfeeds and their sexual or parenting partner, but the parent and the nursling. In antenatal breastfeeding education, we used to describe ideal breastfeeding as being 'on demand'. We have moved away from that language, and we have replaced talking about feeding 'on demand' with 'responsive feeding'. That is partly because the concept of 'on demand' implies baby as boss and does not convey that breastfeeding is a two-way relationship, even from the very beginning. As a baby grows, there are even more conversations about a mother responding to her own needs and her own desires. We should not imply that a 'good mother' switches off her instincts and pushes ahead. We are modelling body autonomy and sharing important lessons about compassion, kindness and patience. But not everything a parent does *has* to have some meaningful lesson for a child. They are asking for kindness for themselves, not just for their child's development. It is rare for a parent to be asked to evaluate how they are feeling about continuing to breastfeed and to check in and make sure it still works for them. We are having more conversations about breastfeeding aversion and agitation, and we are now acknowledging that not every parent universally loves breastfeeding. We also need to make space for the level below agitation, the level of 'I just don't like this anymore'. In the mammal world, we sometimes discuss how mother tigers end up nudging their children off the nipple. That is just as 'natural' as child-led weaning, but we are a long way from recognizing that.

A discussion of weaning older children needs to include an acknowledgement that we are talking about a group of very stressed, and often exhausted, women. Many of those who continue to breast-feed feel socially isolated (Dowling 2018). They may not be open about the fact they are still feeding with their health professionals, nor even their close friends and family. They may be under immense pressure to stop, from people who don't have a concept of what that entails or the role breastfeeding plays in their home and their relationship with their child. The process of weaning isn't simply 'ending breastfeeding', but in many cases, it is learning a new set of parenting skills. Weaning is not just removing something; it is adding a host of new strategies and ways of connecting. Parents may have relied on breastfeeding as the main tool in their parenting tool belt. They may have never dealt with a tantrum or a fall without it. Their child may never have fallen asleep in another way (that late-night drive back from Grandma's being a rare exception). The idea of parenting without the breast can be a frightening concept – even if you know you are ready to stop.

Breastfeeding mothers are under immense pressure to maintain a household even when they return to work outside the home. Recent research suggests that the gap in gender roles is not narrowing as fast as we might hope. When it comes to who does housework in a family where there is a male and female partner, we saw a temporary shift in the early days of the 2020 pandemic, but that was not sustained.

What we saw was that, overall, women's share of housework fell from 65% pre-COVID to 60% during the first lockdown. So, initially, there was a moderate amount of gender rebalancing in the sharing of domestic work. However, by September 2020 the old gender divisions were being re-established. By this point, women were on average doing 62% of housework. (World Economic Forum 2022)

Despite a shift in employment law in many countries, many fathers do not take their full leave entitlement:

The number of countries where paternity leave is enshrined in law has more than doubled to about 90 in the last 20 years; and globally, at least four out of every ten organisations are thought to provide paid leave above the statutory minimum. Yet, the proportion of men who take more than a few days off work when their child is born is tiny. (Cox 2021)

In the UK, the shared parental leave initiative did not produce the expected results:

In 2015, the UK introduced a shared parental leave policy allowing eligible parents to split up to 50 weeks of leave and up to 37 weeks of pay between them. But research in 2018 showed that of the more than 900,000 UK parents who were eligible to take advantage of the policy that year, only 9,200 parents – or about 1% – did. (Cox 2021)

Breastfeeding mothers are isolated, tired and may not know how to start to improve their situation. Sometimes the energy needed to even contemplate a plan feels too much and continuing to suffer seems easier.

Parents are more informed than ever about infant psychology and development and responsive parenting. Even the 'everyday' parenting book discusses neurological development and the impact of the first thousand days of loving care. Parents know that these young brains are their responsibility and take pride in the fact that breastfeeding seemed to tick so many boxes. They are returning to work while still overwhelmed with a feeling of responsibility for their child's emotional welfare. But how does this messaging sit alongside a desire to end breastfeeding a toddler? Parents read about the benefits of continuing to breastfeed and the flood of cortisol that impacts a stressed developing brain, and it is hard to know where to go next. They learn the significance of their child feeling bonded, safe and attached. But what if they want to stop one of their favourite ways of feeling attached? Is it simply a case of deciding to be selfish? A mother centring herself is socially unacceptable and it may be difficult to find information about how to start the process. We have incredibly high standards for what we expect of our society's mothers. They are not only loving carers and providers but also behavioural therapists and psychologists. This is not to imply that high standards and knowledge about the impact of responsive parenting aren't helpful, but let's not pretend modern parents are not under huge pressure in a way the less informed earlier generations may not have been. Ending breastfeeding feels like something parents may want to investigate, but they also feel immensely guilty doing so.

Most of us live in societies and cultures that struggle with endings. As psychotherapist, breastfeeding supporter and doula, Amanda Leon-Joyce (@thedoulamanda), describes:

> As a society, we often struggle with 'good' endings... Relationships end with 'ghosting', or we push people away so that they reject us, and we don't have to take responsibility. We often struggle with death. We need to see weaning as a potential gift for your child's first significant ending in life to be handled well. (Leon-Joyce 2022)

Parents may wean earlier in some cultures because the task of parenting a young child is so thankless. They feel as though they need to regain something and control something; ending breastfeeding feels like the one variable they may as well address, especially when continuing was so poorly understood by wider society anyway. Maybe child-led weaning is more feasible in a world where we feel more recognized and understood and supported. We may find that if mothers are given more space to discuss the challenges and the bad days, continuing breastfeeding feels more manageable. It may be that it feels more achievable to continue if we have permission to say, 'I'm breastfeeding but that doesn't mean I like it every day.' Offering weaning support as a professional includes helping a parent to recognize that they are OK to continue. In my online weaning groups, a significant proportion joined the group expecting to stop but ended up choosing to continue albeit with a greater sense of control over their situation. We can help facilitate that.

We cannot forget the fact that not every mother does get to choose when breastfeeding ends. Not because it is in the hands of a four-year-old being parented in a particular way, but because most women do not get to reach their feeding goals and give up long before the concept of weaning becomes an issue. In the UK, the last published national feeding survey tells us that around 80–85 per cent of mothers who stopped breastfeeding in the first two weeks did not want to stop (Health and Social Care Information Centre 2012, p.82). Of the mothers who had stopped breastfeeding by 8–10 months, over three in five (63 per cent) said that they would have liked to have breastfed for longer (2012, p.106). In a more recent Scottish survey from 2017, 75 per cent of respondents who had stopped giving breast milk to their new baby said that they would have liked to have given breast milk for longer (Scottish Government 2017, p.106). The USA has higher breast-feeding rates and longer duration than most areas of the UK, but the CDC (Centers for Disease Control and Prevention) also acknowledge in their report card that, 'Many families do not breastfeed for as long as they intend to' (2022a, p.2).

We do not know exactly how many parents continue to breastfeed beyond infancy and how many may therefore need support to wean an older baby or child. In many countries, gathering reliable figures for the breastfeeding situation at six months or even six weeks is enough of a challenge. In 2020/21, 21 per cent of Scottish toddlers were still being breastfed at 13–15 months of age (Public Health Scotland 2021). In Australia, the latest figures suggest around 5 per cent are still receiving some breast milk at two years (Australian Breastfeeding Association 2022). In 2018, UNICEF (United Nations Children's Fund) reported a wide disparity in access to breastmilk in low- and middle-income countries: 'Among the poorest families, almost two-thirds (64 per cent) of babies are still breastfed at age two, as recommended by UNICEF and WHO, compared to only 41 per cent among the richest families' (UNICEF UK Baby Friendly Initiative 2018, p.3). However, in high-income countries, we often find the reverse, with less breast-feeding among poorer households. As Shahida Azfar, Deputy Executive Director of UNICEF says, 'We know that wealthy mothers in poor countries are less likely to breastfeed, but somewhat paradoxically, we're seeing indications that in wealthy countries, it's the poor who are the least likely' (UNICEF 2018).

If we are sometimes talking about the more affluent members of society (the ones who accessed support to reach their feeding goals, the ones who were able to make breastfeeding work in family life), that does not mean this is a group any less deserving of our attention, even if the numbers we are talking about are relatively small. Calling for more support for weaning is not greedy. Support for the end of breastfeeding is not a luxury or an extravagance: it's essential. Parents need help to decide to stop and to know how to go about it in a way that is protective of their relationship with their child and the mental health of everyone. The families that do persist with breastfeeding often feel trapped without knowing where to go for support, unlike those who live in lower-income countries where continued breastfeeding is the norm and weaning an older child is also the norm. Ninety-eight per cent of children in western and central Africa are still breastfed at two years (UNICEF UK Baby Friendly Initiative 2018, p.9). Can you imagine the expertise that must exist in every village and neighbourhood when it comes to breastfeeding older children and stopping breastfeeding older children? In contrast there is an expertise desert in most of the communities in which the readers of this book are employed. For many women in western and central Africa, the need for this book would be mystifying. There is an untapped resource when it comes to breastfeeding wisdom and those who continue to breastfeed in high-income countries would benefit from learning from communities where breastfeeding older children is an everyday experience.

If we don't support parents in the end, we create horror stories which reverberate throughout the breastfeeding experience. I have lost count of the times I have heard about a 'sister-in-law' (they can't all be the same one) who 'got stuck' breastfeeding and co-sleeping and bitterly regrets it. I have also come across the parent who is adamant they will end breastfeeding at 12 months to avoid the nightmare of having to wean an older child. It might even be they are reacting to their own experience with their first child. If weaning methods are not discussed openly, parents may be attracted to techniques that clash with the fundamentals of their parenting philosophy, and breastfeeding ends even more unhappily. Supporting breastfeeding without making space to support weaning is like teaching someone how to drive a car, pointing them in the direction of the motorway and neglecting to mention how the brakes work. We have a responsibility. Supporting weaning is supporting women to have agency over their bodies. We cannot talk about abortion rights, rights to contraception and rights to medical care for menopause or endometriosis while ignoring that a woman having a right to end breastfeeding when she wants to is an extension of that same conversation. When babies are first born, we focus on the human rights of the baby and their right to breastmilk. Over time, as nurslings get older, those rights shift and we are talking about a woman's right to have control of what she does with her own body. Supporting mother-led weaning is feminism.

Chapter 2

Making the Decision

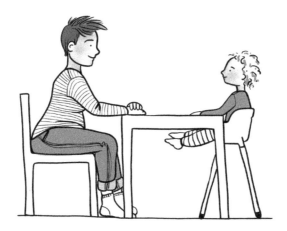

Imagine a parent reaching out for support. Perhaps they fill out a contact form via your professional website. The title reads 'weaning help' and the message says, 'Hi, I'm looking for help to end chest-feeding my 20-month-old son'. What is your next step? You might be setting up an exploratory phone call. You might be arranging a video call. They may be invited to meet you face-to-face. What I hope would not happen is: 'Here's a link to an article about weaning a toddler'. That is sometimes the response we see modelled online and in social media support, and that is understandable when conversations are in public and brief. Peer supporters who spend a considerable amount of time online may absorb that answer as the expected response, but when we are working with parents at a deeper level, we know that is just the beginning of a conversation.

I have been specializing in supporting parents to end breastfeeding for several years. I first wrote a 4000-word article, 'Weaning Toddler Bob and Pre-schooler Billie: How Do You Stop Breastfeeding an Older Child?' (Pickett 2014). This article has been shared in blogs and magazines and many parents discovered me through it and asked for personalized support. I've also focused on weaning on my Instagram account (@emmapickettibclc), interviewing parents and sharing their weaning stories. Since 2020, I have been running peer support groups specifically to support parents through the weaning of older children. The groups meet weekly over Zoom and use WhatsApp for daily support. Currently, about half of my breastfeeding support work is focused on helping parents to stop breastfeeding. I am not explaining all this to talk up my credentials to justify my writing this book. You have it in your hands already now and, presumably, someone paid for it. I want to explain how often parents who come to the weaning conversation *do not end up stopping* – at least not then, and perhaps not for quite some time. I have had entire groups (of around eight members) in which only one mother has stopped breastfeeding by the end of the group (the lifetime of the group is around 6–12 weeks) and the other members were happy with their situation when the group came to a close. After support and discussion, they came to peace with *not* stopping breastfeeding.

When a parent asks for help with weaning, we don't know where they are on a spectrum. They could be at an end that is, 'I've thought about this a lot. I've had support to think about it. I am absolutely done with breastfeeding. I need some information about how to best go about that.' They could be at another end that is, 'I love breastfeeding. I do not want to stop breastfeeding. My child does not want to stop. I just don't like how things feel at the moment. I don't feel I have control of my life. Something needs to change.' Or, 'I have a problem which I don't know how to solve, but stopping breastfeeding might work.' You can see how simply sending someone an article about weaning could be missing the point. It's also true that one article can't do the subject justice anyway, as every family, every parent and every child is unique and have a different relationship to breastfeeding.

So where do we start? We could start by asking a mother how

certain she feels about her decision, and whether she would like to reflect on it further. However, that poses a problem. It may be that she states she is certain she wants to move forward and she does not want any further discussion, but behind that decision, there might be some misinformation. She may have taken the courage to make contact and may have decided she doesn't want to be 'talked out of it'. She could be worried that if we start to ask questions, she may become upset and waver. She may be stopping breastfeeding because she has been told a medication she has to start taking is not compatible with breastfeeding. She may have been told she has to stop to undergo medical treatment. Sadly, time and again, parents are given false information. 'In most cases there are options to support the mother's optimal care while allowing her to continue to breastfeed her baby as long as she wishes' (Jones 2018, p.i). The parents who come across as the most rigid in their decisions could sometimes be the ones masking the most pain.

Some professionals are keen to ensure parents are well informed, like the Drugs in Breastmilk Service in the UK, provided by specialist pharmacists within the Breastfeeding Network and founded by Dr Wendy Jones (the Breastfeeding Network 2019). Professionals and parents can email or message the service through their Facebook page to discuss one or more medications. Other services available include the Drugs and Lactation Database (LactMed) and the InfantRisk Center led by Dr Thomas Hale. Sometimes parents have already said goodbye to breastfeeding in their minds and are shocked to hear that their doctor may not have received accurate information, usually via a manufacturer who is not interested in accepting liability and has not done the necessary trials. Trials cost money, for a start. They may even say a mother has to stop breastfeeding to take a medication because it is not licensed for breastfeeding when the medication itself could be given directly to the baby. We could be at risk of undermining her trust in her doctor at a time when she is already feeling vulnerable, but, hopefully, by providing access to information, we are helping her family and ensuring the doctor's future patients can also make a more informed decision. Sometimes a different medication can be found, the original medication may be safe or breastfeeding need only stop temporarily. Sadly, too often, a health professional who is unaware of the role breastfeeding can play in family life requests that breastfeeding is paused or stopped entirely to minimize all perceived risk, without realizing that stopping breastfeeding brings a different kind of risk.

A mother may be stopping because she would like to get pregnant again and she believes stopping breastfeeding is her only option. The menstrual cycle returns on average at around 14.6 months after giving birth (Bonyata 2018). In most cases, a mother will return to full fertility while she is breastfeeding. However, it depends on the individual and it is difficult to provide any guarantees.

> Some mothers find that once their baby starts sleeping for longer spells at night, or if they are separated in the day time (for instance through the return to work outside the home), this is enough to reduce the effect that breastfeeding has on reducing estrogen levels, so that their bodies can start to menstruate again. Others find that while their baby is still nursing at all, this seems to be enough to suppress menstruation completely. (La Leche League International 2020)

As Hilary Flower, the author of *Adventures in Tandem Nursing*, says, 'tinkering' with breastfeeding patterns may achieve the desired effect, rather than complete weaning (Flower 2018). A menstrual cycle may not be a guarantee of full fertility and may occur without ovulation or with a short luteal phase (a short gap between ovulation and the menstrual bleed, which may not give enough time for implantation to be fully established and to suppress the onset of the next period). A parent needs to learn to recognize signs of ovulation and a book like *Taking Charge of Your Fertility* by Toni Weschler can be helpful (Weschler 2016). If a parent is returning to a fertility clinic for an assisted conception, they may be told that it is a requirement that they end breastfeeding. This can be a painful decision. A parent is giving up something concrete that matters to their current family, for the hope of a future family. A family may feel they must end breastfeeding to maximize the chance of successful conception, but this may not be based on the latest evidence. The Facebook group 'Breastfeeding

Mums Undergoing Fertility Treatment/IVF' can provide a valuable source of support and information. I interviewed its founder, Ali Thomas, for my previous book, *Supporting Breastfeeding Past the First Six Months and Beyond: A Guide for Professionals and Parents* (Pickett 2022), and that interview can be found in Chapter 9: 'Getting Pregnant Again'.

A parent may reach out because they are preparing to return to work and they are finding it hard to imagine combining breastfeeding with their work life. Occasionally, the hope might be that ending breastfeeding will mean a less disturbed night's sleep, so the evidence on that must be shared. In many countries, a parent can return to work with clear laws that protect their lactation, with policies and systems in place. In other countries, mothers returning to work may feel like a pioneer lacking in protection, mentors or a clear pathway. A parent who is preparing for a future return to work needs reminding that the baby in front of them today is not the one they will be leaving. Even just a few weeks might mean a baby will accept solid food more enthusiastically, or nursing patterns may have changed. From as young as eight or nine months old, a baby might not need milk during the working day and can breastfeed when the parent returns home. This connection that comes with feeding, and even complete reverse cycling (where feeding at night is becoming dominant), can come to be cherished by both parties. Older babies can drink water and eat solids when separated from their parents.

Some parents believe that ending breastfeeding will make life easier for those who will be caring for their nursling. Perhaps their child might even miss them less? We need to help them lean into the fact that a well-attached child is going to miss their primary caregiver, whatever is, or is not, coming out of their nipples. The role of the parent is not to sneak away and hope that no upset occurs but to help their child form healthy and meaningful attachments with their new carers and support them through a sense of loss. They will be missed and that is to be validated and understood. A well-attached child will understand that different adults care for them differently: the adults speak differently and help them get to sleep differently; they develop their own caring tools; they may also have been caring for young children professionally for many years. A parent cannot rehearse their child's experience of being put down for a nap by another adult by acting out the part of a different adult. That is an experience that the child and their new caregiver (or perhaps it will be a co-parent) will share between them. If a parent has only limited time at home, it seems a shame to fill the last few weeks with rehearsals for returning to work. It is understandable when there is anxiety about the return to work, but there is a balance between preparation and making the most of the bonding time there is. Breastfed toddlers have been napping happily in nurseries and with Granny, without breastfeeding, since grannies were wearing furs and living in caves (although some of those grannies would also have been lactating – that's a separate conversation).

Sometimes it is grannies and other family members who put on the pressure for breastfeeding to end. In countries and communities with historically low breastfeeding rates, our older population and even the younger parents who struggled to reach their breastfeeding goals, carry a lot of baggage. They may even be traumatized by a sense of failure around their own breastfeeding experience. Of course, sometimes this results in a determination to help the next generation reach their feeding goals but not always. It has been absorbed into the bones of many UK grandparents that a 'good' baby has long intervals between feeds, does not feed for comfort and sleeps independently. When they see a biologically normal baby who is feeding for connection as well as nutrition, and 'breastsleeping' – a term developed by researchers McKenna and Gettler, which describes a phenomenon very familiar to new parents – they struggle (McKenna and Gettler 2016). They may subconsciously, or consciously, feel that their own parenting choices are being judged and prefer you to copy their use of scheduled feeds and bottle-feeding to feel validated. They may have no exposure to accurate scientific information about normal baby behaviour and the value of breastmilk.

Sometimes a wider family may be legitimately worried about a breastfeeding mother. She may be feeling overwhelmed and may even be depressed. Breastfeeding itself may be seen as the cause. As Amy Brown explains in *Why Breastfeeding Grief and Trauma Matter*:

If they just stopped breastfeeding it would all be okay. They'd feel less overwhelmed. Their mental health challenges would magically disappear. All their difficulties were down to breastfeeding and once that was out of the way, they would be fine. Of course, often not much changed when they stopped. The reason so many women were overwhelmed in the first place was that they didn't have support circles around them. Their baby still needed feeding and settling to sleep and now they had lost the mothering tool of being able to breastfeed a fractious baby. And on top of all this, they then mourned the loss of their breastfeeding relationship. (Brown 2019, pp.82–83)

The Drugs in Breastmilk Service can provide information on antidepressants and the continuation of breastfeeding (the Breastfeeding Network 2022) if they may be helpful. Research suggests that mothers who end breastfeeding when they did not want to, and did not meet their feeding goals, are more likely to experience depression and struggle more (Borra, Iacovou and Sevilla 2014). Of course, all that may be true, but a mother suffering from depression can still be someone who wishes to give up breastfeeding. They may have been dealing with pain and challenges, or breastfeeding may have been successful, but they still wish to stop. We will be there for them to make sure breastfeeding ends as safely as possible.

Even when we live in societies where we are more likely to be isolated from wider family, the unsupportive intermittent noise can sometimes grind parents down. Partners may also struggle and be the victim of wider cultural messaging that undermines breastfeeding. Fathers may have limited paternity leave and perceive that breastfeeding is a barrier to them being able to connect with their baby or to do more at night time. It is normal for a young child to develop a bond with their primary caregiver, and removing breastfeeding, with all its benefits for physical and mental health (for both nursling and mother), will not solve the 'problem' and could instead do damage to the relationship between the baby and the mother who is weaning reluctantly. Non-birthing partners may read less about breastfeeding and may not even be involved in antenatal education on breastfeeding. If they are resistant to the idea of feeding an older child, you can signpost them to resources such as kellymom.com or my book *Supporting Breastfeeding Past the First Six Months and Beyond: A Guide for Professionals and Parents:*

Reasons to continue breastfeeding:

- For every 12 months of feeding, there is a 4.3% reduction in breast cancer risk.
- A study of 300,000 women found that breastfeeding reduces risk of heart disease by 10%.
- An Australian study shows that breastfeeding for longer is associated with positive mental health outcomes into adolescence.
- A study in the Philippines shows that longer breastfeeding duration improves social maturity and is associated with better school readiness.
- Continuing to breastfeed reduces the risk of developing type 2 diabetes by 25–47%.
- A 2020 study showed that milk composition from samples at three months and two years were very similar and there was no lost nutritional value. There may even be an increase in fat.
- Some immunological benefits increase in concentration into the second year such as lysozyme, which is a protein that protects against bacteria like E. coli and salmonella.

Continuing to breastfeed beyond two years is supported by the World Health Organization, the American Academy of Pediatrics, the American Academy of Family Physicians and every major health organization worldwide. (Pickett 2022, p.75)

We may like to imagine that if we provide some evidence, then a partner's concerns will melt away and the breastfeeding dyad can continue feeding for as long as they wish. It will rarely be that straightforward. Sometimes prejudices about breastfeeding are deep-seated. Couples may struggle to imagine restarting a sex life alongside breastfeeding. When women sometimes talk about wanting 'their body back', they can mean wanting to feel free to feel sexual and reclaim their breasts as part of their sex life. Many cultures struggle to see lactating breasts as sexual breasts. Women's bodies are compartmentalized.

When a relationship has ended, a breastfeeding parent may be under increased pressure to end breastfeeding by their ex-partner. The organization Breastfeeding for Doctors has produced a useful statement that supports the continuation of breastfeeding:

> In our professional experience, seeking to control or undermine the breastfeeding relationship may be an example of coercive control. Certainly, any attempt to pursue sabotaging the breastfeeding relationship is a direct example of failure to prioritise the best interests of the child and to undermine the primary caregiver's bodily autonomy. It can be triggering for people who did not develop a secure attachment themselves, to witness responsive care and breastfeeding. In the UK, where breastfeeding rates are historically low, professionals may conflate their own cultural biases and opinion with facts. Worldwide, and for much of human history, the average age of weaning has been between two and seven years, with natural outliers beyond this. As with any other developmental stage, like walking or talking, parents can be reassured that weaning will happen in due course without external pressure. Far from being harmful, continued breastfeeding can be part of a responsive, healthy, emotionally secure upbringing. (Breastfeeding for Doctors 2022)

Sometimes mothers want to resume drinking alcohol, taking recreational drugs, or getting a tattoo (many licensed tattoo artists are reluctant to tattoo a breastfeeding parent). They may want to have Botox injections as a beauty treatment. They may wish to do something for themself that they may not want to discuss openly with a breastfeeding supporter.

Sometimes parents are worried that their toddler doesn't seem to be developing an enthusiasm for solid food and they wonder if breastfeeding might be the cause. They may even be advised by others to cut back on breastfeeding to allow solid food eating to develop. Occasionally, when they are particularly worried, they may even wonder if stopping breastfeeding completely is the answer.

Contrary to the common assumption, reducing breastfeeding to create a hungrier child could cause them to be more frustrated at mealtimes. Stacey Zimmels is a speech and language therapist and International Board Certified Lactation Consultant (IBCLC) who specializes in paediatric feeding, and she is the founder of Feed Eat Speak:

> I saw a 12-month-old who wasn't eating any solids beyond a few spoons of prune puree with a lot of distractions. Her mother was returning to work (at home) and in anticipation had reduced daytime feeds to 'help' get her eating. She was feeding her first thing in the morning and then not again until after lunch. It hadn't worked and she was very reluctant to even sit in the highchair at lunchtime. In our first consultation, I suggested reintroducing a mid-morning and mid-afternoon feed so that she was not too hungry at lunchtime. When I reviewed her after a month, her mother reported that by changing the timings of milk feeds she was much happier, she was willing to sit in the highchair for lunch and dinner and was exploring and beginning to taste some finger foods. (Zimmels, quoted in Pickett 2022, p.87)

In a culture that often devalues breastfeeding, ending breastfeeding in order to supposedly improve the intake of solids is a common suggestion. It is sometimes seen as being nutritionally poor, which is far from the truth. We know that if an older child is consuming around 448 ml of milk (which may be the case between 12 and 23 months), they may be consuming only 29 per cent of their energy requirements but 43 per cent of their protein requirements, 36 per cent of their calcium, 75 per cent of their vitamin A, 76 per cent of their folate, 94 per cent of their vitamin B12 and 60 per cent of their vitamin C (Dewey 2001). Sometimes a family may benefit from support in rescheduling how breastfeeding sits alongside feeding solid food, but removing the super food that a child does enjoy seems an illogical response if nutrition is a concern. In the rare case where there is an underlying problem, breastfeeding may go on to have an even greater significance. This idea of stopping breastfeeding to improve solid food intake is an example of a weaning decision that comes from parental desperation. When a parent lacks support, the voices that don't value breastfeeding get louder.

Let's now come at things from a different angle. Rather than the breastfeeding parent either being reluctant to give up breastfeeding, or being someone who is under pressure or the victim of misinformation, let's imagine they *really* do want to stop. In those conversations, we may still have a valuable role in the early stages before we launch into the practicalities. In many cultures, a mother is expected to always put her feelings in second place (or further down the list if more family members are involved). The 'ideal' mother is never angry, always kind and always centres on her child. The 'perfect' mother has time to play, is always patient and, in a breastfeeding context, practises child-led weaning and accepts that her body may not be her own during this phase of her life.

> Mothers today are bullied and guilt-tripped into lowering their sights, reining in their ambitions, shelving their pleasures, and putting their own needs last. It's done explicitly, through guidelines, subtly, through the media and public attitudes, and practically, through structural obstacles at every step of the way. They spend a substantial portion of their waking lives depressed, exhausted and threatful, constantly juggling children's emotional needs, life admin and paid work. Mothers are expected to be responsible and controlled at all times. Yet their dignity and autonomy are constantly undermined. (Glaser 2022, p.267)

When a mother is finding breastfeeding a struggle and wishes to end it, it brings up feelings of guilt and shame. She may be well informed about the value of early attachment and feel that if weaning causes the child distress, it is entirely her fault. She is damaging the child through her selfishness. These feelings can be powerful. Our role can be to help the mother explore where some of these feelings come from and whether they necessarily come from a healthy place. A parent can stop breastfeeding simply because they want to. There is no need to have a reason beyond that or an explanation more complex. We accept that parents may not choose to breastfeed at all. We can accept that they may wish to end at any point. This is about body autonomy.

It may not be possible to eradicate feelings of guilt. However, feelings of guilt about their decision may still be preferable to a feeling of resentment. Psychotherapist Philippa Perry, in her advice column in *The Guardian*, speaks to someone who had to create boundaries with a friend to protect themselves: 'One reader of this column once left a comment saying that if you have to choose between guilt or resentment, choose guilt – wise words. And this is what I urge you to do, choose guilt' (Perry 2022). Sometimes a parent may need to own the fact they will be choosing guilt.

Mothers may have created an image of the kind of mother they wanted to be. They had created an identity of mothering and it only felt complete if they behaved in a certain way and ticked certain boxes. Sometimes parents hold onto behaviours that become part of their identity as a parent. To be *this* kind of parent, child-led weaning feels essential. To centre on their feelings means that identity is being stripped away. In their podcast *Nourishing the Mother*, Bridget Wood and Julie Tenner talk about 'identity crumbling' and 'the shame stumble of the identity crisis' (Wood and Tenner 2022). It is a process of being open to humility and open to re-thinking and saying goodbye to a past version of yourself without shame. It means opening up to a possibility of a future version of yourself. The process of embarking on weaning is often about a mother loving themselves and recognizing when there are feelings of guilt and shame: where is that coming from? Where did that past definition of ideal motherhood come from? Parents may be making choices that feel oppositional to who they thought they were. Parents can ask themselves, 'Did that past self really serve you?' It also isn't about discarding a previous identity but to 'have a sense of integration' (Wood and Tenner 2022) and to say, 'Yes, that was love, and *this* is love.' A parent's past identity led them to where they are now. For some, there will be something spiritual going on. Some parents may even benefit from a process of ceremony or creating a rite of passage to help them say goodbye to that past identity. Parents will be welcoming a future self who has new possibilities.

What is the goal of responsive and kind parenting? It is to help create little people who are empathic and kind and recognize authentic emotions. Psychotherapist Philippa Perry's book *The Book You Wish Your Parents Had Read (and Your Children Will Be Glad That You Did)* has a lot to offer in these conversations. For a start, the aim of parenthood is not to produce a child that is never sad. That is impossible and a dangerous aim. Many of us grow up in families where our feelings were denied as a child, and we may have to work hard to break some ancestral chains. If a parent is metaphorically, or literally, biting their lip to suffer through continued breastfeeding, what are we doing?

> If you're telling lies – or omitting information – to protect children from the reality of the situation, what you are doing is dulling their instincts. You are telling them something different from what they will be sensing and feeling. It won't feel comfortable for them and if they can't articulate that discomfort, it's likely to surface in inconvenient behaviour. (Perry 2020, p.202)

> We owe our children honesty so that means sharing our feelings with them rather than pretending we don't have any. Our feelings and personal preferences inevitably come into a decision like what time they go to bed, and we must not pretend they don't. (p.207)

And whether or not we want to breastfeed, a good parent is an honest and authentic parent who models caring for themselves and expressing themselves truthfully: 'A grumpy honest parent (normally written off as "bad") maybe a better parent than a frustrated and resentful parent hiding behind a facade of syrupy sweetness' (Perry 2020, p.28). Being a good parent is not as simple as minimizing unhappiness whenever possible. Perry explains that the psychoanalyst Adam Phillips said that the demand that we be happy undermines our lives:

> Every life involves pain and pleasure and if we tried to banish pain and drown it out with pleasure or otherwise numb it or distract ourselves, or someone else from it, then we don't learn to accept it and modify it. (Phillips, discussed in Perry 2020, p.75)

We will discuss in later chapters the importance of validating a child's feelings around weaning, and that distraction may not always be a healthy response. We want to support a parent to use strategies that feel as authentic as possible: lack of authenticity 'causes a rupture' in a relationship (Perry 2020, p.230). We create healthier boundaries by describing ourselves and our own needs. We model honesty and self-care. 'The biggest hurdle parents must climb is letting go of the notion that their children should be happy all the time' (2020, p.238). This is true particularly if that happiness comes at the expense of a parent's happiness. We want to give parents space to acknowledge what their true motivation for weaning is. We want them to permit themselves to end breastfeeding for themselves. The relief that can come from that is powerful. It is a necessary step because ending breastfeeding when a child isn't taking the lead requires deep reserves.

If a parent is not sure about their motivation, they are going to be wavering. Guilt and shame may win. Motivations that lack foundation will mean shakiness for everyone. A child that senses confusion is going to feel unsafe. That shakiness is likely to rear its head at 2 am when everything can seem more challenging. When a parent has permitted themself to end breastfeeding, and they understand they have a right to do that, they will be coming from a calmer and clearer place. If instead, for example, they embark on weaning with the justification that this is about improving their toddler's sleep or for 'their sake', they may feel conflicted in the middle of the night when their distressed toddler is doing anything but sleeping and is clearly miserable.

We can help parents to appreciate that the process of weaning is a parenting opportunity. It takes many years for a young child to develop a true sense of empathy. When a child is first born, they don't even realize that they are a separate person. A breastfeeding toddler will usually still perceive their mother's breasts to be their possession. That process of gradually introducing your body autonomy as a parent is a valuable one. In the chapter on setting boundaries, we will explore further how the conversation around weaning will teach the child lessons about their body autonomy.

Ideally, a parent starts the journey of weaning feeling excited about what life might look like on the other side. That's not to say that there won't be some fears and some nervousness along the way, but if we help them to understand their motivations and come to peace with their decision, they will find it much easier to have the strength to support their child through the process.

The role of a breastfeeding supporter is not simply to have that initial conversation, but to walk alongside a parent during the process. Reflection continues throughout. It may be that they feel the need to pause. They may feel as though the balance of their desire to end breastfeeding and the impact it is having on their child feels off-kilter, and their instincts are telling them this isn't the right time. We can help them think through that feeling. Is it coming from a place of guilt (because mothers aren't supposed to prioritize their feelings)? Or does a pause feel like the right thing to do? If so, it is probably fairer on the child for that pause to last more than just a few days, to allow stability to return. A parent may get near to end of the weaning process and realize they are fine to stick with just one final feed, perhaps the bedtime feed. The key is to help the parent find a day-to-day rhythm that works for them. Maybe it wasn't breastfeeding itself that was the primary stress, but the demands of being a parent to a young child who depends on them for emotional support? Adding in new parenting tools, alongside breastfeeding, may mean that breastfeeding can continue happily for longer. A breastfeeding supporter can be the sounding board that helps a parent reach the decision that is right for them.

Chapter 3

Setting Boundaries and Night Weaning

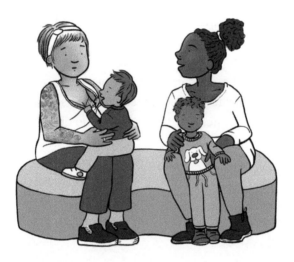

A breastfeeding relationship is two-way from the very beginning. We encourage parents to become confident in reading their babies' feeding cues and to practise responsive feeding, but the parents matter too. They might offer a feed just before they go to bed, or before they have to leave for a nursery pick-up. We don't want them to be in pain – and not simply because it might mean a compromised milk transfer. We don't want parents to be in physical pain, but we also don't want them to be in emotional pain. Sometimes this last concept can get lost in the quest to be a perfect mother who always centres on her child.

As babies get older and turn into toddlers, their needs can sometimes be met in other ways. Breastfeeding might still be a central tenet of the relationship, but parents might also offer a snack, a cuddle, a play session or a book. We don't expect responsive feeding (or what was called 'feeding on demand') to happen indefinitely. We assume parents will work this out for themselves, but I regularly meet kind and loving parents who do not. They struggle to move beyond responsive feeding and believe that it continues to be ideal, even if it doesn't feel entirely comfortable. It doesn't help when a phrase commonly shared in circles that discuss the breastfeeding of older children is 'Don't offer, don't refuse'. A *Huffington Post* article, 'How to Wean from Breastfeeding, According to Lactation Experts', published in October 2022, made it a key focus and described it as 'the "most gentle" method because it "helps gradually wean baby without an abrupt change in routine". But it also takes the longest, so it may not be an option for all parents' (Borresen 2022). It is indeed unlikely to mean an abrupt change in routine but for some parents, change, and the ability to facilitate change, are precisely the point.

If you haven't come across the phrase 'Don't offer, don't refuse', I'm glad because perhaps it is going out of fashion. It's a weaning technique if standing in the rain is a 'washing clothes technique'. You may get there one day, after a long time, but it may not be the most efficient method nor the most practical. It makes me uncomfortable that it undermines the importance of the parent's feelings in the process. It places the parent in an utterly passive role within the breastfeeding relationship and also gives them zero agency over their own body. Even for those who are practising gentle parenting and very much aiming to be child-led, I'm not sure it's an ideal goal we should be endorsing as infant-feeding support professionals. I suspect it was not created by someone who is currently feeding a 23-month-old who asks approximately every 30–40 minutes during a day, including in the supermarket queue, from the back of the car, while you are stir-frying noodles while you are caring for a newborn. I'm not sure if it was created by someone who is struggling with aversion or who is working full-time (or even part-time). Or someone who would like to stop breastfeeding.

Don't offer? Why not? Why can't someone offer when they are

about to go out or they are going to have a bath? Maybe a parent might offer a feed before they have to work or focus on another child. Modelling body autonomy and demonstrating that these are your breasts, and you sometimes get to decide when feeds happen, is a powerful lesson for both members of the partnership. A parent might want to offer because they know that the next hour will be harder, or they prefer to feed in a particular location, or it just feels like the right time. They are taking control of the timing of feeds when it works for them.

Don't refuse. I dislike the use of the word 'refuse'. It's not a word that suggests love and kindness. It implies selfishness and even a bit of brutality. When a parent is simply too 'touched out' to face another feed and suggests a role play game instead, I don't want that to be termed 'refusal'. Every parent, even the ones who don't intend to move towards ending breastfeeding, has a right to decline a breastfeed. What messages are we sending about someone having agency over their own body if every single feed request must be complied with? What opportunities for valuable parenting conversations are we missing? I believe that even the mother who doesn't intend to take any lead over the end of breastfeeding can benefit from sometimes explaining that they don't feel like doing a breastfeed and that's OK. Even if that is met with frustration and annoyance, that is part of honest and healthy parenting. Being a gentle parent means encouraging a child to begin to develop a sense of empathy and start them on the journey of being a caring and emotionally intelligent little person. How can parents do that if they are never allowed to show that their feelings and needs matter too? Many parents describe struggling to find any information about how to wean sensitively beyond 'Don't offer, don't refuse', and they feel judged and alone as a result.

Putting boundaries in place and being honest about how we feel are how relationships work. We should not be endorsing the idea that mothers and parents must always stay silent and compliant. One topic that comes up in breastfeeding older babies and children is nipple twiddling – a nursling feeding while they fiddle with the other nipple. If you spend ten minutes in a social media group where breastfeeding older children is the norm, you'll come across the topic of toddler twiddling. Toddlers enjoy fiddling generally: with the little plastic figure in their hand, the toy car, car keys and glasses. It's how they explore their world, develop their fine motor skills, calm themselves and occupy themselves. And when they are breastfeeding, the other nipple often looks like another appealing button. Some stroke, some twist, some pull, some rub between a finger and thumb, and some twiddle to get to sleep. And the nipple-owner is often struggling.

Imagine if a toddler's favourite thing was fiddling with a parent's eyelashes. Imagine the sticky little fingers and teeny fingernails. Parents would not dream of putting up with that. They might say things like, 'I don't like that. That hurts my eye. That makes me feel uncomfortable. Please don't touch my eye.' Too often, I've seen breastfeeding twiddling tolerated even when it bothers someone just as much. I think because it's the nipple, parents somehow feel as though it's part of breastfeeding. They might read something about how the nursling is stimulating a let-down reflex and think, 'It's natural so I'm stuck'. Or because they can see it gives the nursling comfort and soothes them, they feel obliged to tolerate it.

Often the problem creeps up on a parent. Sometimes literally (with a hand suddenly thrusting down a t-shirt), but I also mean figuratively. It starts when they are small, when it doesn't bother a parent that much, and gradually becomes the norm without a parent ever remembering consenting. Consent is an important word here. I say this a lot when I talk about breastfeeding older children: this is their first intimate relationship. This is a model for how important relationships are going to go in their life and it's about far more than milk delivery and about far more than their comfort. Parents are teaching them slowly and gradually that they are a person too. Child-led weaning is not a scenario where empathy has been removed. Natural-term breastfeeding is not about teaching a child that a parent's feelings don't matter. That would be a waste of a vital life lesson.

An 18-month-old, or even a 3-year-old, is going to struggle with genuine empathy. They are often self-centred in a positive and wonderful way. But how does that phase end? Not by some magical delivery from fairies at around five or six or eight or nine years old. It happens very slowly. Even newborns react to a human face in distress. Day by day, piece by piece, a little brain changes and begins to understand that others have feelings too. Breastfeeding is a wonderful tool for teaching the skills that are at the heart of being a loving human. When you say, 'I don't like it when you fiddle with my other breast', you are helping to make a person who will form healthy relationships decades from now.

Some parents tolerate it because they find a child's distress difficult to cope with and it is easier just to give in. But again, a parent would not tolerate a finger in the eye or something that caused physical pain and damage. Just because an experience is in the sphere of breastfeeding, it does not mean the only person that matters is the nursling. A parent can offer some alternatives. They can tuck a piece of cloth, or something textured, into their clothing and encourage fiddling with that as an alternative. They could offer an alternative nipple shape – perhaps a knitted breast or even a silicone one. A parent can move their child's hand to a different place with a gentle and repetitive phrase and be consistent. They could let them say one 'hello' to the nipple and then give them a choice about where the fiddling will continue: 'Do you want my bra clip or your nose? Do you want red flannel or shirt button?' On a practical note, once nipple twiddling ends and a parent feels more comfortable, this means more oxytocin and milk flow and an improved breastfeeding experience for all.

Other nursing manner problems can include 'gymnurstics' – a toddler moving their whole body while breastfeeding. They might be attempting to stand while still being attached to the breast. They might be twisting round to try and see something while feeding. Or a child might ask for a feed by pulling at a parent's clothing. That might initially seem cute, but it could wear thin if a parent is in a public place or a feed isn't comfortable at that moment. These kinds of battles are a way to rehearse the bigger conversation. When a parent permits themself to say no to nipple twiddling or an uncomfortable position, it is a way to practise the larger conversation that comes later when parent-led weaning happens. They realize that they can stay consistent and, even after some initial distress, a nursling will respect the boundaries and accept them if a parent remains clear and firm. Distress and annoyance are something that their child will survive. We want our children to live in a world of authentic emotions and to model honesty. As Naomi Aldort says, in *Raising Our Children, Raising Ourselves*:

Telling your child that you 'feel fine' when you are ready to explode teaches them to suppress or hide strong emotions. In addition, left to imagine why you are upset, your child, being self-centred by nature, is likely to either assume it is because of him, conclude that one has to be dishonest when feeling bad or come up with some other life-draining interpretations. (Aldort 2005, p.154)

We are not simply encouraging a parent to model emotional honesty. This is also an opportunity for important conversations about body autonomy and consent. When little people go out into the world, we want them to develop respect for the body autonomy of others. This includes not bashing another child over the head at the sand tray at the nursery when a favourite truck is taken. It also includes harder conversations about having the right to feel safe and to speak up if someone touches them in a way that doesn't feel comfortable.

In the UK, the NSPCC (National Society for the Prevention of Cruelty to Children) has its 'Talk PANTS!' campaign (NSPCC 2012). It is aimed at children aged roughly 5–11 years old and the aim is to introduce a foundation for open conversations about body autonomy. PANTS is an acronym: 'Privates are private. Always remember your body belongs to you. No means no. Talk about secrets that upset you. Speak up, someone can help you' (NSPCC 2012).

The campaign uses phrases like, 'Your body belongs to you. No one should ever make you do things that make you feel embarrassed or uncomfortable,' and, 'You're in control of your body and the most important thing is how *you* feel. If you want to say "no", it's your choice.' Now let's imagine a parent trying to teach a child these concepts while gritting their teeth through nipple twiddling and tolerating their nursling pulling aggressively at their clothing. If a parent is struggling to permit themself to self-centre, they will perhaps be more open to seeing these conversations as a source of learning and modelling for their child. As Sarah Ockwell-Smith reminds us, compassionate parenting doesn't mean always letting your child control their world entirely:

Compassionate respectful parenting is mindful always of the

importance of attachment and the parent–infant dyad; however, it never prescribes that parents should always let the child get their way, and never suggests that children shouldn't be set firm boundaries. (Ockwell-Smith 2013, p.174)

Our toddlers need to experience disappointment to learn that sometimes they must put the needs of others first. (p.176)

Setting limits around nursing can mean that breastfeeding can continue for longer in many cases. Some parents consider ending breastfeeding entirely when they are struggling with nipple twiddling or aggressive requests for feeds. They may find that by putting boundaries in place, their child not only learns valuable lessons about treating others that can make breastfeeding more manageable, but also feels safer within themself. Lawrence Cohen in *Playful Parenting*: 'If children are not provided with firm, clear limits, they end up feeling either omnipotent or out of control. Neither of those is real confidence' (Cohen 2012, p.249).

Those who continue breastfeeding beyond infancy are often dedicated to a kind of parenting which centres on the emotions of their child and is about love and connection. This can be a reaction to the authoritarian parenting they experienced during the last decades. However, it is important to emphasize that a loving compassionate parent is a parent who can say no, and a relationship is stronger as a result. Boundaries that matter are enforced with love and respect. Good parenting is not about avoiding upsetting a child at all costs:

Those who parent with compassion and respect are not afraid of making their child cry in attempting to reinforce important limits; they are strong enough to cope with the resulting strong emotions that will surface in the toddler. (Ockwell-Smith 2013, p.176)

If a parent is struggling with nursing manners, this matters. It is not something that they have to tolerate just because it only lasts a few minutes, or it won't last forever. The conversation is an opportunity to practise communication and honesty that will take the relationship to a new level and prepare for later conversations.

For many families, the process of parent-led weaning begins with night weaning. This is by no means universal. Many of us will have met the breastfed five-month-old baby who sleeps through the night, for no obvious reason. Some children will night wean themselves in infancy, much to the dismay of other parents who continue to experience regular night wakings and requests for night feeds for years. Parents are quick to blame themselves if their child continues to wake regularly. They often imagine that they must have done something, even if they have no idea what and no sense of how things could have gone differently.

It is worth starting a discussion on night weaning by reminding parents that if regular night waking isn't causing them distress, it does not mean something has to change. As Lyndsey Hookway, sleep expert and International Board Certified Lactation Consultant (IBCLC), reminds us:

> Most books seem to assume that all children under five will sleep from 7:00 pm to 7:00 am. I hate to break it to you, but not all children sleep like this. It's also a culturally incompetent idea to assume that all children (or adults for that matter) work steadily towards monophasic sleep. (Hookway 2021, p.9)

Some parents believe they must embark on night weaning because it will improve their toddler's sleep. Lyndsey Hookway again:

> I am often asked if toddlers will be sleep deprived if they wake up frequently at night. It sounds logical, doesn't it? After all, if someone wakes us up 4–10 times per night, we feel very tired the next day. But is it the same for our little ones? Well – it depends... If your child wakes and needs something from you to go back to sleep, then as long as they get what they need promptly and return to sleep, no – they are not sleep deprived. In my experience we often assume our little ones are tired or even exhausted because *we are*. We assume our toddlers need an early night or a longer nap because *we need those things*. But

remember that fragmented sleep is not the same as sleep deprivation. (Hookway 2021, p.24)

If a parent wants to night wean in the hope it will improve their own sleep, that is a valid motivation in itself. However, night weaning may not immediately improve their sleep as young children may continue to wake up, and getting them back to sleep may be trickier without breastfeeding. Night weaning because someone feels unwell or has reached a crisis point is unlikely to be helpful. The process of night weaning will initially take more effort and energy. If a parent feels they are in crisis, they will ideally get support from other adults to help them get to a place where they then can start night weaning.

Where might a parent start? There are limited resources online and some parents will find themselves using controlled crying or leaving their child to 'self-soothe' without support. When a parent chooses to use a non-responsive strategy, with a previous history of responding to their child at night and breastfeeding between sleep cycles, it often comes from a place of desperation. When parents have breastfed beyond infancy, it is rarely a first choice. The evidence around the risks of sleep training methods is mixed, but most professionals who work closely with new families don't see a lack of conclusive proof of harm as a sign there should be no hesitation. As Lyndsey Hookway puts it:

> In the context of what we know about responsive parenting, attachment, attunement, and relationship building, as well as the uncertainty we have about individual children's responses, and their internal vulnerabilities and resilience levels, it's not something I personally am willing to take the risk with, which is why I continue to advocate for responsive sleep support. (Hookway 2021, p.43)

What are some approaches to night weaning an older nursling? For younger babies, you will be substituting a breast for a bottle. That isn't going to be the recommendation for a toddler, not least because bottles aren't recommended beyond 12 months, but also because the desire to breastfeed at night time is often not about the milk itself. That is not to say it is not a factor at all. Some toddlers are thirsty at night, and some may not eat a significant amount of solids during the day and rely on overnight calories to keep them going. This might mean having a cup of water on hand at night, in a way a parent didn't previously, or reflecting on daytime feeding and trying to realign the day/night calorie balance. For older nurslings, we are starting with an assumption that we are usually talking about the breast being a source of safety and comfort and a way to settle between sleep cycles.

How quickly can the process of night weaning happen? Dr Jay Gordon describes it as possible to night wean in just a matter of days. In his article 'Sleep, Changing Patterns in the Family Bed' (Gordon 2020), Gordon assumes co-sleeping is the natural state of affairs. He suggests a parent start by choosing their core seven hours of sleep, for example, 11 pm to 6 am. This is the time when parents will try to change patterns. For the first three nights, if a child wakes before 11 pm, they breastfeed back to sleep as normal. However, within those core hours, a parent begins by nursing but then leaves the child awake and they are settled to sleep using another method.

Dr Gordon prepares parents to anticipate an angry response:

> Now, he will tell you that he is angry and intensely dislikes this new routine. I believe him. He will also try to tell you that he's scared. I believe he's angry, but a baby who's had hundreds of nights in a row of cuddling is not scared of falling asleep with your hand on his back and your voice in his ear. Angry, yes. Scared, no, not really. (Gordon 2020)

A nursling has to fall asleep to then be able to breastfeed again. Gordon then suggests that for the second set of three nights, there is no nursing on waking and another settling method is needed. Following that, the settling method is toned down, until less and less parental intervention is needed.

This sounds prescriptive, and at first glance, it is. However, Gordon does remind parents:

> If, at any point, this is feeling 'wrong' to you, stop, wait some months and start over. Don't go against your 'gut instincts' which tell you that this is the wrong time to get longer sleep intervals from your baby.

Your instincts are better than any sleep-modification program ever written. (Gordon 2020)

The faster method may be useful for parents who are weaning quickly because of a family emergency. This method can also be valuable for parents who don't have a partner or a support network and are at breaking point. What I do appreciate is that Gordon is giving parents permission to care for themselves and saying that they matter too. In reality, parents may choose to go slower and insert some additional steps if that is possible.

There may be some barriers to this method within some families. Some nurslings fall back to sleep so quickly on the breast that a parent does not have time to remove them and try to settle them in another way. Some children may be confused about why night feeds happen sometimes and not at other times. They may not understand that 10.55 pm is acceptable and 11.03 pm is not. With an older nursling, you may be able to explicitly explain your approach and even show the hours on a clock. With a younger child, that is not going to be possible. A parent may decide that the confusion is too much and they need to have a consistent approach that lasts all night.

A child who has never experienced any limits around breastfeeding may get quite a shock to the system and they may do better if there are some boundaries in the day, even if daytime weaning is some way off. It might be useful to introduce the concept that 'boobies are tired' or 'Mummy is tired and boobies need a rest too'. It can be easier first to introduce limits at a time when the parent is awake, calm and in control, as the middle of the night can be a difficult starting point for everybody.

During those first three nights with the Gordon method, it is quite a big ask for a child with no previous experience to fall asleep without the breast. They had one habit that worked well, and that they loved, and now it is gone and they do not know what to do. They no longer feel safe, and they are a long way from feeling soothed. Plus, the person who has done this to them is offering cuddles and hugs and they may feel angry towards that person, and hardly in the mood for a cuddle.

What can be helpful is the concept of habit-stacking (a term used by Lyndsey Hookway). We want the child to have more than one association with safe and soothing bedtime and the process of falling asleep. Then as the breastfeeding is removed, they are left with something familiar that already helps their brain to think, 'Ahh, yes, sleep time now'. After all, being a creature of habit is a normal human state of affairs. Adults would also not be thrilled if our familiar routine was yanked out from under us overnight. Parents can introduce one or two additional habits alongside breastfeeding. It is something that involves the parent, so they are still offering co-regulation once the breastfeeding finishes. It will differ for every child. Some would be irritated by stroking or patting and may prefer something auditory. A parent might choose a gentle phrase that can be repeated. They might tell a narrative along the lines of, 'You are sleeping now. Mummy is sleeping now. Granny is sleeping now. The cats are sleeping now. The birds in the trees are sleeping now.' You can see how this one goes, and it can be expanded or contracted as needed. When it later comes time for night weaning, the parent can add in, 'Boobies are sleeping now'. Some families might choose gentle singing or a white noise machine with ocean sounds. There is something to be said for having a recording of the 'sleepy story' on a parent's phone that can be played at 2 am when the parent is at breaking point.

For older nurslings, guided meditation can also be a valuable tool at bedtime and the peaceful language repeated during the night in smaller chunks. An older child may be able to express an opinion on what they would like to use as their additional sleep habit. At the same time, it can be useful to have a conversation during the day about the process of falling asleep, to help reinforce that this is a process that involves an element of choice. How does Daddy fall asleep at night? How does a friend? What do they do when they can't fall asleep easily? A parent might role play falling asleep with cuddly toys during playtime. What is Teddy going to choose? And teddy might be angry with Mummy because booby isn't happening throughout the night. A parent might play bedtimes, where they are the child and the nursling becomes the parent. Or original roles might be maintained, and the parent offers alternatives to the breast. Role play can be a useful way to work through emotions.

Breastfeeding toddlers often haven't attached to a cuddly toy at bedtime. Why would they? The parent is their cuddly toy. However, it might be useful to introduce a transitional object, to provide one further means of support if night weaning is going to happen. Again, with an older nursling, this is something they may like to have agency over. A parent might explain that one day boobies will go away and they can choose a new friend to be with them at night to help them.

A floor bed as a base for the child is a useful tool when a parent is preparing for night weaning. I don't feel it is realistic when a parent imagines that a toddler who has previously breastfed at night and co-slept is about to accept a move back to a cot. Sometimes parents imagine that the closeness has been the 'problem'. Perhaps if the child is moved into a different room and is physically separated, they won't sense the parent or 'smell the milk'. A cot might be the answer. That ship is likely to have sailed. For an older child who has not had the continuity of a cot being their safe space, a later introduction is unlikely to be accepted peacefully, and we want this process to be peaceful where possible. Inserting a physical barrier, alongside the removal of the breast, is likely to reinforce the fear of loss and isolation. Night weaning is going to be hard work for a parent. A floor bed aids their sleep, as well as their child's.

In the nights before the onset of night weaning, a daytime conversation is valuable. This is not something that comes out of the blue. However, weeks of preparation are unlikely to be helpful. Being gentle is not always the same thing as being *very* slow. A young child is unlikely to have a sophisticated sense of time, and concepts like 'next month' or even 'next week' are fairly meaningless. Something like 'in a few days' might be more useful. A parent might discuss it on the bus, walking back from the park or at dinner time. A parent will eventually remind their child that, 'Tonight is the last night that booby happens all night. Then tomorrow booby is sleeping at night.' Or they might say, 'tonight is the last night booby happens all night. Tomorrow, we can only do two boobies at night.' They remind them that it will be hard, and they will be there to help them. Then the morning before the big night, there are lots of reminders. Picture books can be a helpful tool in this discussion, and you can read more about the options in Chapter 7.

What is important to emphasize is that a parent will be there to support the child, whatever they are feeling. We are not implying that we are asking them to be a 'good boy' or to 'try hard'. Equally, the next morning, we are not praising them for not being upset. All feelings are welcome because the child is loved unconditionally. Parents are not praising a lack of emotion. Just as we don't praise a child who doesn't cry when they are in physical pain, we are not going to praise a child who doesn't show distress when they experience emotional pain. It usually works well if the bedtime feed remains, although a parent may choose to end it slightly before the child is asleep. As has been the case for a while (potentially weeks), the bedtime feed is accompanied by other familiar sleep habits.

How fast the next stage goes will be very individual. An older child may comprehend a transition where they are only allowed two feeds at night (or one) and the rest of the time they need to go back to sleep in a different way. They may also understand that they can have milk but only for a few seconds – perhaps 'count to ten' or 'count to five'. This can help both the parent and child to feel as though they have agency over the situation. Other children do better with a clear message that there is no milk until morning, and overnight the breast is not available. Some children will not understand partial night weaning and get stuck in negotiation mode. I often speak to parents who feel that their child will manage better with full night weaning alongside loving support, which happens abruptly after a phase of habit-stacking, as opposed to removing night feeds one-by-one. It is still 'gentle' because it happens alongside emotional support and understanding and with preparation.

However fast or slow a parent goes, their child may have an emotional reaction. The parent is there to support them through it, which is not the same thing as trying to make the feelings go away. Lyndsey Hookway says:

> You don't need to make the tears go away. Expressing emotion about this change is normal and understandable. It's not your job to erase the emotion or distract your child from it, but to acknowledge that it's hard for your child and provide emotional scaffolding through it. (Hookway 2021, p.269)

This is the key message of parent-led weaning, whether night weaning or full weaning. If a child has had a normal relationship with the breast and a healthy attachment to the parent, this will be a loss. They were not ready, even though the parent was. Parent-led weaning is not a process of pretending the child was ready. It is the parent acknowledging that they weren't, that they are going to need help, that they are going to feel sad, and that it is still OK for the parent to proceed under those circumstances. Other family members must be on board with this message. We don't ask if a nursling was a 'good girl' at breakfast or tell someone they are being 'so brave' about night weaning. We don't offer reward charts or give treats for the repression of emotions. All emotions are welcome.

There are likely to be three or four nights that are very hard for the parent. All their feelings of guilt are going to surface. This doesn't feel like something parents are supposed to force on their child. This is why spending time reflecting on their motivation and owning their decision is so important. A parent who starts night weaning with the belief that this is 'for their toddler' is going to crumble quickly. A parent needs to know why they are doing this and that they have permitted themselves to do this for themselves. As Dr Jay Gordon says:

> Your toddler is aware that you are right beside him, offering comfort and soothing. It just isn't the mode of comfort he wants at the moment. It is hard to listen to him fuss, but it will work. I believe that a well-loved baby, after a year or more in the family bed, will be the ultimate beneficiary of his parents getting more sleep. Not coincidentally, the parents benefit 'big time', too. (Gordon 2020)

Parents may find that a child appears to be accepting new methods of co-regulation and settling, and then there is a difficult night that appears to come out of the blue. A child who is not settling after more than a week probably needs more support and consolidation of the new methods. It may be that there are other factors affecting their sleep pressure and their ability to return to sleep.

What about the breastfeeding parent going away and sleeping elsewhere to facilitate night weaning? Can they go away for a few nights and let the partner take the lead? We will discuss this further in the chapter on partners, but I have a feeling you know what I am going to say here. Of course, a parent would choose to avoid seeing their child in pain if they could. These are often parents who are very tired and very desperate. They are only human. It sounds appealing to imagine they can go away for a week or less and, when they return, the situation will be fixed.

There are two main problems. First off, it often doesn't work. A toddler may be at the age where they are very conscious of separation and trust issues. When they are finally reunited with the breastfeeding parent, the relationship has been ruptured and repair is needed. What is good for repair? More breastfeeding! I have heard multiple stories of mothers being leapt on when they return home and breastfeeding continuing with a new level of enthusiasm. After a few difficult nights, a parent is not back to square one but is at square minus five. Second, it is simply avoiding a conversation that needs to happen. This conversation cannot be avoided. This is an opportunity for learning and supporting a child through a difficult change. These emotions have to be confronted head-on and the child needs the milk provider to demonstrate, 'I am not leaving you. Only the milk is going. This is not a loss of *me*. This is the loss of just one aspect of me.' When a parent leaves the home, the child is losing the whole parent and that can be terrifying, even if a loving partner is there to offer them support. For the child, this is not merely separation, it is desertion. The breastfeeding parent needs to develop a new parenting tool belt and that takes practice. We will talk more about how a partner can support in Chapter 8.

So, after weeks of habit-stacking and days of preparing and warning, the parent finally stops night-time breastfeeding. As mentioned, there may be a difficult few days. Some children will struggle for longer than others. A typical scenario is three or four nights that are very challenging before things start to get easier. There may be an occasional relapse if a child is unwell or when the realization that the change is going to be permanent suddenly hits a new level. If a parent instinctively feels this isn't going in a comfortable direction, they may decide the process needs to be paused. This isn't giving in or behaving inconsistently. This is being a responsive parent. However, it is probably not wise to restart just a few days later. The process needs evaluation and reflection.

If sleep is a particular area of struggle for a family, it may be valuable to look beyond night weaning and seek support from a professional sleep consultant first. This is not the same thing as a 'sleep trainer', and the ideal person will have an understanding of normal sleep patterns and the significance of parent/child attachment. In the UK, a good place to start is the holistic sleep coaching community, where parents can be reassured that professionals are trained to understand responsive parenting. Many lactation consultants have gone on to do holistic training, to sit alongside their work as a breastfeeding support professional. You can read more about the underpinning philosophy in Lyndsey Hookway's book, *Holistic Sleep Coaching: Gentle Alternatives to Sleep Training for Health and Childcare Professionals* (2018). In other countries, parents can find professionals who offer support on sleep who also understand the value of natural-term breastfeeding and understand how night weaning and night-time feeding sit alongside other factors, but it may take some investigation.

Chapter 4

The Effect of Weaning on the Parent

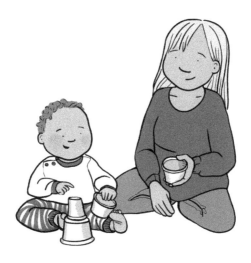

When breastfeeding comes to an end, it affects everyone. A family will need to develop different routines and other ways to express affection. There is a new language of connection and comfort. It's a different world. For many parents, there is an enormous sense of relief. However, even for the parents who were single-minded in their determination to end breastfeeding, there may be some emotional and physical effects that they need to be prepared for. There is a tricky balance between informing parents and frightening them to the extent that they worry that they may not be able to cope with the fallout. Truthfully, most people are not emotionally affected in a negative way by the end of breastfeeding, but enough are that it is useful to discuss it and give some warning. It can be reassuring to parents to know, for example, that a period of feeling emotionally flat may be hormonal and natural, and not their body telling them to restart breastfeeding because they have made a horrible mistake.

Whether someone will feel a physical impact at the end of breast-feeding is going to depend on what the level of milk production was at the point of stopping, as well as their own breast texture and level of glandular and fatty tissue. If a baby was entirely dependent on breastfeeding for their nutritional needs, and a parent was producing perhaps 800 ml in 24 hours, that production needs to wind down slowly. This is one reason we discuss taking a minimum of three to four days before dropping another feed. Breasts are likely to fill with milk and become engorged, and engorgement can be painful and distressing. As the milk storage areas fill, breasts are filled with blood and cell-tissue fluid. The grape-like lobules in the milk storage areas can feel lumpy under the skin and this can be frightening for a parent who has spent months, or even years, associating lumpiness with blocked ducts. It is natural to assume that lumps must be massaged away or removed, but this may not be possible and shouldn't be the aim. Milk storage areas that remain full are doing some important jobs. As the prolactin receptors in the alveoli remain distended, the prolactin hormone can't lock in to send more signals to increase milk production. The whey protein known as FIL (feedback inhibitor of lactation) also accumulates, which sends signals to slow milk synthesis. Fullness is therefore part of the natural process which slows milk production.

However, this is a balance, and we want the reduction to be as comfortable as possible. Breasts need to be well supported. Pain relief may be helpful, which might include an anti-inflammatory such as ibuprofen, provided there is no medical reason it can't be given. Cool compresses, and even raw cabbage leaves, may also provide relief. Cabbage leaves have long been known to be a tool for relieving engorgement, although convincing research to prove this may be lacking (Wong, Koh and Gail 2012). One study did find that cabbage was more effective than cool gel packs in the relief of engorgement post-partum (Wong *et al.* 2017). Cool compresses are likely to reduce blood flow and promote lymph drainage. The Academy of Breastfeeding Medicine, in their 2022 Mastitis protocol, states:

> Ice and nonsteroidal anti-inflammatory drugs (NSAIDs) can reduce edema and inflammation and provide symptomatic relief, and acetaminophen/paracetamol can provide analgesia. For example, ice can be applied every hour or more frequently if desired. Ibuprofen can be dosed 800 mg every 8 hours and acetaminophen/paracetamol 1,000 mg every 8 hours in the acute setting... Sunflower or soy lecithin 5–10 g daily by mouth may be taken to reduce inflammation in ducts and emulsify milk. (Mitchell *et al.* 2022)

Issues are going to be similar when we are talking about severe engorgement in the absence of mastitis. Applying ice directly to the breast is not ideal and using a pack of frozen peas wrapped in cloth is often suggested by breastfeeding supporters.

In some cases, where a parent is struggling with continued lactation, herbal or pharmaceutical options may be considered. Many of the dopamine agonists used to cease lactation have high-risk side effects and are rarely used, but may have a place in an emergency, and breastfeeding supporters can refer to doctors for prescribing. Bromocriptine or cabergoline are two options. Both have significant side effects but cabergoline is usually considered to be the preferred option (Johnson *et al.* 2020). Other options (also outside the remit of most breastfeeding supporters) include pseudoephedrine: 'Pseudoephedrine is a non-prescription decongestant medication that can decrease milk production, although the mechanism of action remains unknown. Aljazaf and colleagues found that a 60 mg dose decreased milk production by 24%' (quoted in Johnson *et al.* 2020).

Contraception containing oestrogen can also reduce milk supply. There are herbal options too: 'Peppermint, sage, jasmine flowers, and chasteberry commonly have been used to reduce milk production' (Johnson *et al.* 2020). Scientific studies are lacking, though. Kelly Bonyata, IBCLC (International Board Certified Lactation Consultant), describes a process for using sage:

To use dried sage (*Salvia officinalis*) for reducing milk supply, take ¼ teaspoon of sage 3 × per day for 1–3 days. You can mix the sage in vegetable juice (for example, V-8), but it won't mix well into other juices. You can also mix it into other foods or a broth. If you don't like the taste of sage, try putting it into a tiny piece of sandwich and swallowing it whole – peanut butter or something else a bit sticky seems to work best for holding the sage in place. Tear off the corner of the sandwich containing the sage (it should be a very small section) and swallow it without chewing (that's why you need a very small section).

To use sage tea for decreasing milk supply, infuse 1 tablespoon of dried sage in 1 cup of boiling water. Steep for 5–15 minutes. Drink 1 cup, 2–6 times per day. You can use a tincture of sage instead: 30–60 drops of tincture, 3–6 times a day. Do not use sage essential oil – it should not be taken internally. (Bonyata 2023a)

These recommendations assume a parent is managing hyper-lactation, and if full weaning is taking place, technically there would be no limits on amounts, other than what someone's palate can cope with.

Nancy Mohrbacher describes some other approaches recommended by different authors: Winema Wilson Lanoue advocates reducing salt intake alongside wearing a firm bra and other measures. Kathleen Huggins again suggests wearing chilled cabbage leaves, replacing them with fresh leaves every three to four hours. She also describes taking 100mg of vitamin B6: two pills three times a day 'for the first day and one tablet daily thereafter; possible side effects include nausea, vomiting, diarrhea, and dark, yellow-coloured urine' (Mohrbacher 2020, p.178). However, this dose contradicts information given elsewhere and this level is sometimes suggested to treat vasospasm rather than reduce milk supply. The InfantRisk Center (who specialize in medications and lactation) say online, 'Vitamin B6 has been associated with seizures (rarely) at doses of 300mg/day or more. Also, vitamin B6 decreases prolactin levels at doses greater than 600 mg/day, which would likely decrease Mom's milk supply' (Pride 2011).

The main message to parents is that the ultimate method to reduce milk supply is to stop removing milk. That means patience. We know that involution (the termination of milk-producing cells) can take at least 40 days and some parents report drips of milk continuing for a surprisingly long period. There is a wide range of normal: 'Small amounts of milk or serous fluid are commonly expressed for weeks, months or years from women who have previously been pregnant or lactating' (Wambach and Riordan 2016, p.95). It can be tempting to test and see if milk is still present, but of course, every test is interpreted by the body as a request for more milk.

When might we worry? If milk production continues over an extended period despite no stimulation or surges post-lactation, we would encourage a parent to speak to their doctor to rule out hormonal issues or other breast health concerns. If a localized firm area in the breast becomes especially tender and if a parent starts to feel generally unwell, with flu-like symptoms, we may have to consider the possibility of mastitis. If a parent has a pale skin tone, we may see areas of redness on the breast. Sometimes a parent may need to take a step back from weaning until mastitis is resolved. That doesn't always have to mean a resumption of breastfeeding if expressing can be effective. Some parents prefer to slow the process of reducing milk production by expressing milk between the dropping of feeds. Expressing can be reduced even more gradually and over a longer period. This might be easier to manage than communicating with a reluctant nursling. If a parent has a history of blocked ducts or mastitis, they may be especially nervous about weaning and may want to use herbs or medication. It is not recommended to bind breasts during the weaning process as that can increase the risk of blocked ducts, nor should a parent restrict their intake of fluids.

If mastitis does develop and is untreated, or insufficiently treated, a parent may be at risk of developing an abscess. When there is a bacterial infection, a localized self-enclosed pocket of pus may develop, which can require draining either through incision or a needle aspiration under ultrasound. Depending on the location, an abscess can present as an unresolved blocked duct and levels of pain can vary, so any firm area not resolving will need investigation.

When do breasts 'go back to normal'? This will also have some individual variation. In one study, 'By 18 months postpartum, lobular area content and lobule composition were indistinguishable from nulliparous cases' (Jindal *et al.* 2014). It may be that older mothers who are perimenopausal or menopausal do not see breast texture returning in the same way. However, research shows it is not breastfeeding that affects breast shape in the long term, but pregnancy and weight changes (Pisacane, Continisio and the Italian Work Group on Breastfeeding 2004).

What about the emotional impact of weaning? There is a huge range of experiences. Sometimes the physical is tied up with the emotional. Parents describe struggling with breast symptoms but also other physical symptoms that appear like PMS (premenstrual syndrome). Yet other physical symptoms could be explained by hormonal changes or the body reacting to a big life change. You won't be surprised to hear that research is lacking in this area. Some parents don't seem to feel any impact of weaning. It may be easier when the ending is gradual and the milk supply has diminished over time. Here is Rhiannon:

I actively encouraged snacks rather than feeds until we got down to around four feeds a day (around 16 months). From there she dropped feeds organically, just stopped asking until we were on morning and night. My little one has always had a bottle of cow's milk at night since a year; sometimes when I'm on a long shift, with her Dada ... at about 19 months she began to ask for 'bot nuk' at night time rather than me. I continued to feed her on waking in the mornings (a glorious, relaxing morning routine). From around two years she began not asking every morning, and from 28 months she stopped asking (possibly due to changes with me being pregnant again, but we haven't made a big deal of that with her). I haven't felt huge hormonal changes really, and now, although sad that it has come to an end, I'm so chuffed with all we achieved following a pretty tough Covid-baby-bugger-all-support start.
(*Rhiannon*)

Others struggle considerably more. Sara weaned at 18 months:

I was an emotional wreck for a couple of weeks; instead of baby blues after birth, I had a boob-blues. I was in an oxytocin high for such a long time and the hormone readjusting combined with the physical pain hit me hard. Everyone was telling me I should feel relieved that he was the one who decided to wean, and I know breastfeeding is a two-way relationship (I know all the theory), but I did feel sad and rejected for a while and also frustrated because not many people seemed to understand while I was feeling like that.
(Sara)

Grace, after 25 months:

I had really low mood and actually ended up speaking to my GP about this who reassured me it was normal. I missed our closeness and worried I couldn't parent without breastfeeding; it was such a big part of our relationship that I struggled for a good two months to adjust physically, emotionally and mentally. I'm so proud of our journey and never imagined how far we would get! He had adapted so well to stopping, especially at bedtime, but even now I still miss it sometimes.
(Grace)

Gillian (her nursling was just under two years old):

For the first week, I felt really resentful towards people who had negative views towards breastfeeding. I felt quite bitter towards their views and very emotional – yet I'm normally a very calm person. It was almost like everything that I had bottled up came out and I felt angry about how little that people understand about the benefits of breastfeeding, yet also how hard it can be and how difficult it is to wean a toddler. Physically I suffered symptoms of PMS and felt like I was ovulating for three months before I had my first period. *(Gillian)*

Sarah's breastfeeding journey ended after 34 months:

Physically, I experienced swollen breasts and clogged ducts and the very unexpected hot flushes in the middle of the night! I felt all kinds of emotions; happiness seeing how my little one had developed such confidence from our journey, but also a feeling of loss, which was probably due to my child being fine with the change. Feeding to sleep turned to bedtime cuddles, which I was thankful for as I'd got to the stage of beginning to feel 'touched out' at the 'neediness' and not being able to pass part of bedtime routine to my partner. My hormones seemed to be all over the place for a few weeks, with lots of weeping episodes that I hadn't really experienced since the early postnatal period. I look back on our experience fondly and am happy that we ended our journey at the right time for both of us! *(Sarah)*

Grace weaned during pregnancy at three years and nine months:

As it was very gradual for the both of us, it didn't have the emotional fallout that it potentially could have had, if ended more abruptly. He cuddles my chest and rests his head on my breasts sometimes when he wants to be close so we both get that closeness, which is lovely. Emotionally for me, it was fine because it was gradual, and I could see it coming and I made my peace with it. It was a beautiful experience. I also think hormonally I didn't get any side effects of it ending because it was gradual. There was also some overlap at the end of breastfeeding with pregnancy. I asked him if the milk had changed or whether it was still there, and he always said yes that

he was getting it. So, I don't know whether that had any impact. I feel very lucky and content with how breastfeeding ended for us and it's something I will cherish forever.
(Grace)

However, gradually weaning doesn't seem to have a protective effect for everyone. Katie, who weaned at three years and one month:

Just because it's been a very gradual process doesn't mean that I haven't experienced breastfeeding grief. I've felt pretty emotional. Breastfeeding has helped me parent through allergies, silent reflux, numerous illnesses and when my daughter broke her leg – I've been so grateful for my boobs! This phase of parenting coming to an end I feel is something wider society should recognize and acknowledge as important to so many people, however long or short their journeys are.
(Katie)

Rachel's story highlights why support for ending breastfeeding is so important:

I heard from a friend that going 'cold turkey' had worked for a friend of theirs. In desperation, myself and my wife committed to going for it. I left for the weekend, stayed at my parents and she and her mum supported our son through it. I was initially relieved. I slept, rested and was away for three nights. The physical impact was painful, with engorged breasts. But the emotional fallout was absolutely horrendous – I've never experienced grief like it. It consumed me intensely for a week and eased somewhat for a few more weeks. I cannot recommend weaning this way; I feel like it was the most brutal way to end such a special and irreplaceable bond between us. Even though I 'chose' it, I really didn't realize the detrimental impact it would have on me emotionally. I can only assume the confusion and distress it caused my son and the guilt I feel from that is nearly unbearable. Although my son now sleeps through the night, we both miss breastfeeding so much.

I wish I could have kept day feeds and worked out some way to night wean. I really feel that I tried to explore ways to make it work but it feels very much like there is so little practical support around stopping or reducing breastfeeding. Especially when you get past a certain point – people made out that I should be glad 'I made it this far', but with better support, I feel I could have continued day feeds.

My main message is that stopping suddenly felt like the only way but actually it was, on reflection, the worst way to get what we needed – more sleep. This way created a hormone storm, on top of intense guilt and grief, and I would never recommend it: I wish I'd known another way.

(Rachel)

Some parents struggle with a sense of rejection they weren't anticipating as they navigate a new relationship. Jodie, who weaned at 15 months:

I was an emotional wreck when I weaned my first daughter. I felt like I had lost my superpower; the boob was the answer to everything. When I stopped breastfeeding, I actually had to parent her now and work out what is wrong.

I was very hormonal, I cried a lot, but my daughter wasn't even bothered: she never asked for it again. Two weeks after I weaned her, she was having a tantrum and I still had some milk; I tried to breastfeed her and she looked at me with disgust: 'Why are you putting your breast in my mouth?'

I weaned slowly so it wasn't traumatic for her, and I didn't get engorged, but I never considered how it would be for me emotionally. I was so upset to have stopped but I was desperate to get

pregnant again. I had my first ovulation a week after I stopped breastfeeding and got pregnant.
(*Jodie*)

Some parents are just not quite ready and struggle when a child leads the weaning process, as Libby's story demonstrates:

It was the height of the pandemic – June 2020 – and my daughter decided she was done with breastfeeding. Never had I wanted her to have breastmilk more than [at that moment] as this seemingly unstoppable virus raged. The end was gradual: when I reflect on probably the last six months prior, it was me initiating the majority of the feeds, initiating them because I was used to the daily rhythm we had carved out for ourselves. She had dropped the feeding-to-sleep association herself long before, but that last bedtime feed was still part of our routine. And it got shorter and shorter and shorter until one day my husband gently put a hand on my shoulder and said, 'Do you think she wants that feed still?' 'Of course!' I replied. This was my boob-obsessed, bottle-refusing baby who had fed every one-and-a-half hours on the dot as an infant. She couldn't possibly not want to breastfeed any more at just 2½ years old… could she?! The thought settled with me for a few days. And these were the scary days of lockdowns, sanitizing food packets when they were delivered, daily press conferences and scary statistics. I'd taken great comfort in the fact that my dear daughter was still having breastmilk to help protect her. But it kept nagging me, and the feeds by this point were seconds, maybe a minute long. So, one night, I just didn't offer. We still did our full routine, I just waited for her to initiate the feed. She would surely – but she didn't. And this continued on for about five days. Me waiting. Her not asking. She was done – she hadn't mentioned it at all. I was shattered. I thought we would continue until at least three, probably much beyond. Gone was my reassurance of my secret weapon against the pandemic. And how on earth did you parent without breastfeeding?! That was the biggest for me, and for about six months after, when she hurt herself or needed regulating – I wished we were still feeding. Oh, the hormone slump! As a trained feeding supporter, I knew it was coming – but wow! The feelings of rejection that she had chosen to stop...and the hormone shift was huge. It was like a fog for a couple of weeks, and then it lifted. She asked to latch about three weeks after stopping and I obliged, but she had lost her latch. She asked me to tell her what to do, but she couldn't. Hers was more curiosity; she wasn't upset in the slightest, just exploring. I now reflect back and am so grateful our journey gently wound down, on her terms. No big emotions for her, no big dramas, worries and having to implement changes. She just stopped when she wanted, which was a promise I'd made to her when we were still in the hospital after her arrival – we would keep going with feeding for as long as we could.

(Libby)

Some parents report changes to their skin such as an increase in acne. Others describe hair shedding as being more noticeable. It's hard to know what to attribute to the end of breastfeeding, as hormonal shifts are happening throughout this period and oestrogen levels rise. Our job is not to try to second guess the cause of symptoms but to offer information, where it exists, and empathy.

A key point is that parent-led breastfeeding, and a parent who is desperate to end breastfeeding, may still experience some sadness and should be prepared for the possibility. Christina, who weaned at 22 months:

Even though it was a decision I made, I distinctly remember when the realization hit me that I'd breastfed for the last time. I cried uncontrollably for an hour or so, then slowly started to make peace with the loss I had suffered.

(Christina)

Sometimes when parents have embarked on parent-led weaning, they feel embarrassed when they experience mixed emotions. It can almost feel as though their brain is betraying them: 'Surely, if we are putting our child through all this, the least we can do is feel certain about our decision.' Parents need to allow themselves to feel all the feelings, just as they first permitted themselves to lead on weaning. As IBCLC Glenni Lorick says, 'This is the first weaning' (Lorick 2009), but parenting is a series of weanings as our children gradually become more independent and move into the wider world. Ending breastfeeding can feel like a symbol of us mattering less. It's interesting how parents react differently to milestones being reached. Some parents feel nothing but pride and satisfaction, but I have also known parents to get tearful when a birthday is reached. Some feel emotional when solid food is started, as it feels like a form of letting go. Breastfeeding has been an enormous part of their life. It may be one of the achievements that they feel most proud of, especially if they have persevered to make breastfeeding work in the face of insufficient support. Few of us live in communities where we perform rites of passage or ceremonial activities, but they can have an emotional purpose. A parent who has led the weaning process has just as much right to celebrate and mark their achievement in breastfeeding. This might include ordering a piece of breastmilk jewellery, planting a special plant or just a moment with friends and family.

For some parents, there can be a feeling that an entire community has been lost. Daily social media interactions may have involved the breastfeeding and chest-feeding community and feeling part of a team. Their membership in the team will always be needed, and the breastfeeding world depends on peer supporters to help families that are waiting in the wings.

Even when a mother has met her breastfeeding goals and is choosing to end breastfeeding, the emotional after-effects can be profound. For a deeper exploration of feelings of grief around breastfeeding, focused on women (who wanted to breastfeed) stopping before they were ready, I recommend Amy Brown's book *Why Breastfeeding Grief and Trauma Matter* (Brown 2019).

Chapter 5

Weaning under Twelve Months

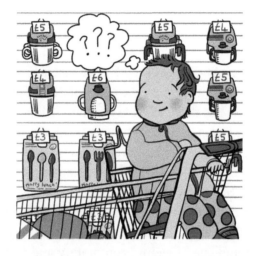

As breastfeeding supporters, our mission is to support a parent to reach their feeding goals. It is not always the case that we can fly the flag for breastfeeding advocacy in every conversation we have, even if we might want to. We have conversations about combination feeding. We talk with families about introducing a bottle of formula, when there is no medical reason for doing so, but simply because they want to, and they've asked about it. There will certainly be a place to discuss the reasons why continuing to exclusively breastfeed is ideal, and we might go into some detail in doing that while also discussing how to protect the breastfeeding that will remain, but we provide the information the family is asking for. We respect the choice of the parents and if we are not capable of doing that, we are in the wrong line of work. We have to make sure we never lose sight of the fact that we are centring on the families we support, even if their parenting choices don't fit with our philosophies or even the basics of scientific evidence and research. It could mean taking some deep breaths.

One of the hardest aspects of working in this field can be supporting families who are surrounded by cultural noise that can be anti-breastfeeding and normalizes feeding of formula. It can also be challenging to support families who perceive breastfeeding as simply a milk delivery system, or when a parent is under pressure to return to work in a setting where their lactation will not be supported. We accept the realities that are presented before us and support parents to be the parents they need to be within that reality. All infant feeding specialists can support with bottle-feeding, although some have less experience than others. There is sometimes a myth that midwives and professionals trained by the UNICEF Baby Friendly Initiative (BFI), or working in BFI-accredited settings, are 'not allowed' to talk about bottle-feeding and formula use. This is simply not the case. On the UK BFI 'About' page:

> We also support parents who are formula feeding by providing information on choosing milks and making up feeds, helping them to feed safely and responsively. In addition, we advocate for better regulation of marketing of breastmilk substitutes so that health professionals and families can receive scientific, unbiased and factual information about infant feeding. (UNICEF UK Baby Friendly Initiative 2023a)

The aim is to support all parents to develop close and loving relationships with their babies and to give babies the best possible start in life.

Is it comfortable when a mother who is breastfeeding a six-month-old baby says they feel 'touched out' and they want to stop breastfeeding? Is it easy when a mother contacts us to say that breastfeeding a ten-month-old is quite long enough and she now needs help to ensure breastfeeding has completely finished by 12 months? In the early days, it can be harder to separate our understanding of what breastfeeding really is and what it can offer from the information the parents we support need from us. You may occasionally come across a breastfeeding supporter online, or in real life, who continues to struggle with that separation.

'Lactivists' are often perceived as militants who judge parents and push their views about breastfeeding on others, even when it doesn't support the parent's situation or needs. Mercifully, I've never met anyone who fits that description in real life. As a volunteer with the Association of Breastfeeding Mothers in the UK for over 15 years, and on the National Breastfeeding Helpline, I'm glad to say I've also never met one who has undergone training in breastfeeding support in the UK who struggles to focus on the parents' goals.

When you speak to parents every day, you understand that choices around infant feeding are rarely simple. Often, the choice is removed entirely by a baby who struggles to latch, has physiological barriers to effective feeding (such as tongue tie) or a parent who has not had access to effective breastfeeding support, nor support from friends and family. There may be factors that we never understand and cannot fix – mothers who have a relationship with their breasts and their body that are a barrier to breastfeeding; partners and grannies who put pressure on mothers to stop (and we can't fix that with our counselling skills); employers who have no interest in facilitating expressing breaks. In the UK, the right to express milk in the workplace and maintain breastfeeding is a grey area and not as clearly protected as it is in so many other countries. We might be talking to an autistic parent who has struggled with the intense physical experience of breastfeeding and is now at a point where they must move on to feed their child in a way which will hopefully be less of 'a sensory nightmare' (Professor Jane Wilson, quoted in Zia 2022).

And of course, a mother may want to stop breastfeeding because she simply does. She doesn't have to be under pressure or have a profound psychological barrier or a practical hurdle she cannot overcome, even with support. She might just want to stop. She doesn't need a lecture on the value of continuing to 12 months and beyond. If she were to receive that without invitation, the chances are she would not be returning for support in the future with her next child, nor signposting any friends and family in our direction. We want a world where parents can breastfeed for as long as they want to. We want them to be fully informed and supported and we want them to be able to make choices for themselves. Countless parents don't get to choose to breastfeed for as long as they want, and they need our focus. When we meet the mother who is well informed and determined to stop, we don't want her to feel for a second that we are offering judgement. Devoting energy to attempting to change the mind of someone who is confident in their decision to stop is a misunderstanding of what breastfeeding support should be. Recommendations around breast-feeding are on a population level. That doesn't mean that they work for every family and every parent and in every context. As Professor Amy Brown says to parents: 'You don't have to justify your decisions, and certainly not to people who haven't been involved in creating and caring for your baby' (Brown 2021, p.286).

That means that we don't offer judgement, not that we are faking it. Breastfeeding counsellors need to be authentic and genuine and empathic. When we develop our listening skills and centre ourselves on the families we are supporting, that will hopefully come naturally. If you feel you are struggling, it is important to acknowledge your bias, forgive yourself for it and actively seek to overcome it in your conversations with families. Breastfeeding support can be an isolated profession and it can take conscious effort to make sure you have a network that can offer you supervision and a listening ear.

As an IBCLC (International Board Certified Lactation Consultant) in private practice, you might develop a peer network where you can reach out. As a volunteer, you should have a supervisor who supports you to explore your feelings and reflect on your triggers. You might have a journal where you confidentially reflect on why a particular client or family is a particular challenge, and that may include reflect-ing on your own feeding experience, or that of someone close to you.

Let's imagine we receive a call from the mother of a six-month-old baby who wishes to end breastfeeding and we are arranging to give them support. We may ask some initial questions about moti-vation, and we will do so calmly and efficiently. We do not want to give the impression that we are speaking from a place of needing to be convinced that her decision is justified and that she has 'earned' our support. How does she feel about her decision? We might say, 'Tell me about how you reached your decision,' or, 'Tell me about the background to your decision,' rather than, 'Why do you want to stop breastfeeding now?' Those first few seconds of conversation, the language you use and your tone, will give her important messages about what she can expect. Let's not shy away from stating it: a mother who is asking for support to end breastfeeding under 12 months probably understands that she is stopping sooner than the World Health Organization and her local breastfeeding support team might dream. She is possibly holding her breath a little in trepidation, wondering if she is going to have to justify her decision and what our response might be.

Does she need to start a particular medication? And is she fully informed about its compatibility with breastfeeding? Is this about a return to work, and does she understand what the practicalities of a return to work while breastfeeding can look like? She may perceive that she has to provide 30 ml of expressed milk for every hour they are separated, when an older baby may manage with less, alongside solid food and some extra feeds at night. She may not be aware that her supply could adjust to allow for some breastfeeding alongside the use of formula. Is her motivation related to a desire to return to full fertility? Does she know that it is perfectly normal for her menstrual cycle not to have returned at six months? She might not realize that it is possible to return to full fertility and conceive while still breastfeeding. She also may not be aware of the research around optimum child spacing, which currently suggests that at least an 18-month gap between births reduces risk (Schummers *et al.* 2018).

Is she motivated by a belief that not breastfeeding will improve her baby's sleep? We can provide useful information that will help her to be fully informed. Research suggests that when babies are 6–12 months, the introduction of formula and moving to formula feeding does not reduce night wakings.

Of infants in this age range, 78.6% still regularly woke at least once a night, with 61.4% receiving one or more milk feeds. Both night wakings and night feeds decreased with age. No difference in night wakings or night feeds was found between mothers who were currently breast-feeding or formula feeding... Breastfeeding has no impact on infant sleep in the second 6 months postpartum. (Brown and Harries 2015)

Her baby is likely to continue waking and may need a bottle through the night, as night feeds continue to be normal. They may fall asleep easily after a bottle, or they may miss the sleep-inducing hormones. She may also miss them, and it may take her longer to fall asleep in between feeds. If breastfeeding is otherwise going well, and the only aim is to reduce night wakings, we need to direct her to more reading and ensure she has realistic expectations. It takes skill to explore a decision without giving the impression we are aiming to talk her out of it. Let's not forget that our literal job title often implies we are on the side of breastfeeding. It is completely appropriate to be up front about that reality. Why not say, 'I know I am a breastfeeding counsellor/lactation consultant, but my job is to support you to reach your goals.' Or, 'How confident do you feel about your decision on a scale of one to ten?' Or, 'Would you like some information to help you explore your decision?' We want to help a mother to future-proof her decision. We do not want her to return in a few months to say, 'Why didn't you tell me that my baby's sleep might not improve?' because we were keen to ensure we were supportive of her decision and not appearing to be judgemental.

Let's imagine we have helped her to reflect on her decision and she is informed and confident and now keen to move forward. Let's assume that she is looking to move to formula feeding and not feed her baby her own expressed milk. She will need some information about the starting of solid food. If her baby has not yet started solid food, it's important she understand that it may be weeks and sometimes months before solid food quantities reach a sufficient level that milk can start to be less of a priority. It is not until 12 months that solid food provides more calories and nutrients than milk. We have a long time of focusing on milk, and solid food is only gradually moving from the experience of experimenting with tastes and textures to something more substantial (First Steps Nutrition Trust 2015).

A baby of around 7–9 months who is taking solid food reliably will still need around 600 ml (20 oz) of formula in 24 hours (NHS Better Health Start for Life 2023). From around 10 to 12 months, if we can assume that solids have become more established, we're expecting still around 400 ml (13 oz) of formula (Brown 2021, p.205). If a baby is under six months and relying entirely on milk for their nutrition, we usually expect them to have around 150–200 ml of formula per kg of their body weight in 24 hours (NHS 2019). That is a big range, and we will discuss later the importance of practising responsive bottle-feeding and allowing the baby to communicate their needs and their appetite. With breastfeeding, the volume of milk intake does not vary between around six weeks and six months. That's often a shock to parents who expect the volume to keep going up and up as their baby grows. When breastfeeding, babies send signals and vary fat levels and nutritional content themselves, and breastmilk is very bioavailable. With formula, we are going to need more volume to keep meeting a growing baby's needs.

Under six months, a bottle will likely be the most effective way to feed a young baby. But it's not imperative. Some babies with special needs may be fed in different ways; some babies may be able to feed effectively from a cup. However, in the vast majority of cases, a bottle will be efficient and allow a caregiver to hold a baby and connect with them during a feed and to minimize waste. Ideally, the transition from breastfeeding to exclusive bottle-feeding happens gradually. A parent has been producing a full milk supply and it is going to take time for their body to get the message that the request has changed. If that isn't handled carefully, at the very least we could be looking at engorgement and blocked ducts. In more serious cases, we could be increasing the risk of mastitis and abscesses, as discussed in Chapter 4.

There are physical adaptations that are needed but also emotional ones. If a young baby is feeding roughly eight times in 24 hours (it could easily be more), then we would start by looking at the formula total needed over 24 hours and divide by eight. Let's imagine we are supporting a four-month-old baby who weighs 7 kg. That would give us an intake of around 1,050–1,400 ml of formula in 24 hours (150 ml × 7 as a minimum, 200 ml × 7 as a maximum). As someone from a breast-feeding support background, let's pause for a moment to consider:

that feels like a lot of liquid! We're used to an intake of 600–800 ml of breastmilk for a baby exclusively breastfeeding (Bonyata 2023b). There is a huge range when babies are breastfeeding, but 1,400 ml would not be a normal volume of consumption. We need to be careful we don't immediately set up an expectation that will mean stress for both baby and parent. There is a little stomach and digestive system here that is going to be dealing with a new kind of milk, with new proteins, new ingredients and the development of new bacterial flora. If we start with 1000 ml of formula in 24 hours, at eight feeds, that's around 125 ml in each bottle. However, this is not a race. If day one means one bottle of 30 ml of formula at some point in the day (perhaps before a breastfeed), when everyone is in a good mood, that is a good place to start. If that volume increases gradually until one feed is entirely with the bottle, we might then pause for a couple of days to let breasts adjust and to consider the next steps. Dropping one breastfeed no faster than every three days feels sensible.

What kind of bottle is best? Parents often get pulled down a rabbit hole when it comes to this question. If a family is ending breastfeeding, we have less need to consider which bottle is closer to the breast or protective of breastfeeding. We are looking for a bottle which is affordable, easy to buy where a family lives and with replaceable teats that are also easy to find. What about the speed of flow? If a baby has been breastfeeding, they may have been dealing with a faster milk ejection reflex and been gulping away, or they may have grown accustomed to a steadier flow. It seems sensible to start with the lower-flow teats if a parent is not sure what is best. Those are the teats that either describe themselves as being for newborns or are size 1.

Truthfully, most families who are ending breastfeeding have already been mixing feeding and have had some bottle experience. They may already have a bottle that works and a brand of formula they prefer. Choosing a type of formula for the first time is another rabbit hole. In the UK, as in other countries where the 'WHO code' or the International Code of the Marketing of Breastmilk Substitutes was adopted into law, or partially adopted, infant formula brands cannot be advertised to families. In the UK, this applies to first infant formula for newborn to six-month-old babies. However, follow-on formula (for babies aged six months plus) is advertised and on television so those brands often seep into the consciousness. The UK charity First Steps Nutrition Trust, an independent evidence-based organization that provides information on all aspects of early nutrition, explains the situation:

> Despite regulations saying that the label text, images and colours should differentiate follow-on formula from infant formula and for infant milk marketed as foods for special medical purposes, manufacturers continue to use similar product designs and colours, with the brand the biggest feature of the product label. This enables them to cross-brand products and allow the advertising of follow-on formula to influence families in their infant formula choice. (First Steps Nutrition Trust 2021a, p.2)

When should a family use first infant formula and when should follow-on formula be used? First Steps Nutrition Trust explains:

> Follow-on formula is unnecessary (WHO, 2013). The NHS is clear that follow-on formula should never be fed to babies under 6 months and that there are no benefits to switching to follow-on formula after 6 months, with infant formula recommended throughout the first year. (First Steps Nutrition Trust 2021a, p.1)

There is also no evidence to support the use of a formula designed for 'hungry babies', which contains more casein protein as opposed to whey protein and may slow digestion but not provide more calories (Banks 2022, p.67).

In some countries, we deal with more blatant advertising or even samples being offered to families. Throughout the world, companies are reaching out to professionals whether through sponsorship of events or providing 'product information'. Even where advertising is apparently regulated, the law may not be enforced and social media is particularly slippery with influencers and bloggers promoting products and being seen by new and vulnerable families. Parents are inevitably going to be influenced by friends and family too. This is not surprising when 'parents can feel very lonely and unsupported when making choices about infant formula and bottles' (Banks 2022, p.15). If they are asking for information on what type of formula is best, the answer is straightforward – that we are unable to answer. That isn't just because it compromises us professionally, but because it is not possible to answer.

> All infant formulas have to be of a similar composition to comply with UK compositional requirements and all brands are nutritionally adequate for infants. If a substance was found that was definitely beneficial for infant health that could be added to infant formula, it would be in all infant formula by law. (First Steps Nutrition Trust 2021b, p.8)

That needs to be explained sensitively, to ensure we don't give the impression that breastfeeding supporters aren't allowed to talk about 'evil' formula or that it doesn't matter because 'it is all rubbish'. It does not matter because the law says that when something is discovered to be essential for babies, everyone has to include it in their ingredients. The psychology behind parents' purchasing choices is complex, and buildings full of professionals devote their lives to analysing motivation. The message that a family may as well buy the cheapest formula, such as a supermarket's own brand, and not the most expensive in the luxurious packaging (which has possibly paid for better placement on shop shelves) can be hard to absorb. One benefit of coming from a breastfeeding support background is that we are not perceived to have a horse in this race. Hopefully, the reality that the most expensive is not the best will be understood. Families who have previously breastfed may be more vulnerable to messaging that non-cow's milk formula is 'better'. In fact,

> Infant formula made from goats' milk has to have the same amino-acid composition as infant formula made from cows' milk, and there is considered to be no difference between first infant formula made from cows' milk protein or goats' milk protein in terms of their allergenicity or their digestibility (EFSA, 2012). It is important that health

professionals are aware that goats' milk-based infant formulas are unsuitable for infants with cows' milk protein allergy. (First Steps Nutrition Trust 2020, pp.1–2)

Soy-based formula is not recommended under six months and there are even concerns for babies older than six months. First Steps Nutrition again:

Soya-based infant formula is not recommended for use in infants under 6 months of age, and in infants over 6 months, it should only be used under medical supervision. This is for several reasons:

- Children are as likely to be allergic to soya protein as to cows' milk protein.
- Soya is a rich source of phyto-oestrogens and these mimic sex hormones in the body. For older children and adults, some soya is not a problem, but for babies under 6 months who have soya protein-based infant formula as their sole source of nutrition or older infants who have high volumes of milk, current guidance in the UK is that the phyto-oestrogens in soya-based infant formula should be carefully considered as a risk.
- The carbohydrate source of soya protein-based infant formula is maltodextrin, which has a greater potential to damage teeth than the lactose in infant formula based on cows' or goats' milk. If infants are allergic to cows' milk, they will be prescribed a suitable infant formula by their GP. (First Steps Nutrition Trust 2021b, p.11)

If a cow's milk allergy is suspected, a parent will need to speak to their doctor. They may be offered a formula with a hydrolysed protein or one that is amino-acid based. This decision will be made after a proper diagnosis and full investigation. Some brands are vegetarian, but the majority of infant formula brands are not. Fish oils are often used, and animal rennet is used in the process of separating whey and casein. In the UK, there are currently no vegan formula brands available, even when the protein in the milk is plant-based, as micronutrients can be animal sourced (such as vitamin D from sheep's wool).

A vegan family wishing to end breastfeeding is going to be reliant on donor human milk and realistically this is going to be unscreened informal milk sharing. Only at 12 months might a vegan milk alternative be suitable alongside solid food. If a family is going to be giving a young child a vegan diet, they will be well informed about nutritional needs, and First Steps Nutrition Trust's resource aimed at vegan families is a useful overview: *Eating Well: Vegan Infants and Under-5s* (First Steps Nutrition Trust 2014). I should mention here that no one should ever attempt to make their own formula, whatever blogs with beautiful photographs and snazzy design may suggest to you. Some contain levels of vitamin A, protein and iron that are harmful to babies (Banks 2022, p.124). After six months, when a baby is eating solid food, they can still be in danger if their milk increases their risk of infection and malnutrition. Families with a history of breastfeeding may be tempted to look for ways to avoid giving their money to formula companies, but other than donor human milk, there is no alternative milk suitable under 12 months. Cows' milk as a main drink for a young baby can be dangerous. The CDC explains:

> Before your child is 12 months old, cows' milk may put him or her at risk for intestinal bleeding. It also has too many proteins and minerals for your baby's kidneys to handle and does not have the right amount of nutrients your baby needs. (Centers for Disease Control and Prevention 2022b)

So, we have a bottle, and we have a brand of formula. We need to make sure families understand how to prepare a bottle safely, especially if they are using a formula for the first time. Powdered formula is not sterile in manufacture and that means we need contact with recently boiled water to kill any bacteria it may contain, and thoroughly wash hands, surfaces and equipment. Liquid ready-made formula is sterile but the cost of that means it is extremely unlikely a baby consuming more than 500 ml a day is going to be taking ready-made formula exclusively. Ready-made formula can cost 60p per 100 ml (UK), compared to 27p for 100 ml of the same brand's powdered formula (First Steps Nutrition Trust 2022a, pp.9–10).

A kettle filled with at least one litre of fresh tap water needs to be boiled and left for no longer than 30 minutes so it remains at 70 degrees Celsius or above. Then water is put in a sterile bottle and powder is added using a level scoop. If smaller quantities of water are being boiled, it can only remain in the kettle for much shorter periods before combining with the formula as it will cool more quickly. (A larger quantity of water will hold its temperature for longer). Bottled water may contain too much sodium or sulphate (First Steps Nutrition Trust 2022b, p.32). It seems that 70 degrees precisely may not be hot enough as the water will rapidly cool once added to the bottle (First Steps Nutrition Trust 2022b, p.9). The powder then needs to be mixed by shaking, although Shel Banks IBCLC suggests this might add air bubbles, which could later cause wind, and advocates swirling or mixing with a sterile spoon (Banks 2022, p.94).

Then the milk will need cooling and the temperature tested on an inner arm/wrist before being fed to a baby. This is a major expedition for a family used to just unclipping a bra. There might be a temptation to skip a few steps. When a family has been used to handling breast-milk, with its antibacterial properties, they might not even have been sterilizing a breast pump. Microwaves are not recommended to heat milk as they can leave hot spots. It can be useful to store boiled water in a thermos flask, to avoid having to boil a kettle each time. Some machines use a small quantity of boiled water to mix with the formula, before then adding cool water to deliver a bottle at room temperature. There are significant concerns this might not be sufficient to reduce the risk of bacterial infection (Grant, A. *et al.* 2023).

The Foods Standards Agency in Ireland is an example of one agency that does not recommend their use due to insufficient evidence about their safety (Food Safety Authority of Ireland 2021, p.38). There are also some concerns about the ease of cleaning the machines (Banks 2022, p.49).

When a bottle has been made-up, it needs to be given within two hours if it is being stored at room temperature (First Steps Nutrition Trust 2022b, p.8). Of course, all this assumes that a baby is happily taking a bottle. For a family who wants to end breastfeeding, moving to the bottle may not be so easy. Some breastfeeding supporters are contacted by parents who are desperate for their baby to start drinking from a bottle, but their baby did not receive the memo. This can be distressing for a parent who feels trapped, and distressing for a baby who starts to sense the tension and desperation. Breastfed babies are used to being in charge.

We want all bottle-feeding parents to be confident with a technique known as responsive bottle-feeding (sometimes referred to as 'paced bottle-feeding'). We know that bottle-feeding may increase the risk of overeating and obesity (UNICEF UK Baby Friendly Initiative 2023b). It seems logical when we consider that formula milk doesn't contain a hormone like leptin that appears to have a protective effect against obesity (Palou, Picó and Palou 2018). In addition, when a baby is feeding directly at the breast, they work increasingly harder as the milk slowly increases in fat content and requires more effort to remove. The mother's milk ejection reflex slows. That slowing process gives them more time to develop a feeling of fullness and a baby can move into non-nutritive sucking if they wish, without being overwhelmed. They can also choose to detach whenever they wish.

At the bottle, none of this is straightforward. With younger babies, the sucking reflex will kick in automatically when a teat makes contact with the palate, and they will automatically swallow when liquid reaches the back of the mouth. The sucking reflex will have faded as a baby gets older and is moving from breastfeeding to bottle-feeding, but it may require more effort for a baby to signal they wish to stop feeding, and that indication may come late. With responsive bottle-feeding, we are giving the baby a better chance of being in control. It is not completely protective of overfeeding, but it may help. We want to encourage parents to continue to respond to their baby's cues, rather than move to timed and scheduled feeds. A feed is a time for connection and communication. We always knew breastfeeding was more than just a milk delivery system and a bottle feed can also be an opportunity for closeness. Not everyone who has chosen to move away from breastfeeding is doing so with complete joy and certainty. A parent who has made a choice voluntarily and confidentially may still be nervous about how their relationship with their baby might change. As Shel Banks says in her book *Why Formula Feeding Matters*:

'Understanding and applying responsive feeding principles can minimise any feelings of loss of relationship when breastfeeding is not happening' (Banks 2022, p.13).

The way we hold the baby and a bottle may also reduce the chance of overfeeding. UNICEF UK explains:

> Hold baby close in a semi-upright position so you can see their face and reassure them by looking into their eyes and talking to them during the feed. Try and alternate the side you hold baby. Begin by inviting baby to open their mouth: softly rub the teat against their top lip. Gently insert the teat into baby's mouth, keeping the bottle in a horizontal position (just slightly tipped) to prevent milk from flowing too fast. Watch your baby and follow the cues for when they need a break; these signs will be different from one baby to the next, they may splay their fingers and toes, spill milk out of their mouth, stop sucking, turn their head away or push the bottle away. Gently remove the teat or bring the bottle downwards to cut off the flow of milk. (UNICEF UK Baby Friendly Initiative 2019)

Some parents are concerned about the idea of bringing the bottle downwards as they are focused on the possibility of air getting in and the baby being windy after a feed. But a feed that is too fast, with a flow a baby can't cope with, or doesn't want, is also going to mean air getting ingested as the suck/swallow/breathe pattern is disrupted.

Sometimes when a parent sits a baby more upright and starts to invite the baby to show interest, the baby will start to consent to receive the bottle. We want to encourage their natural rooting reflex by touching their lips with the bottle teat. The first move is not to try to simply 'put the bottle in'. If the baby is still resisting, what else might help? Sometimes, it might be a good idea to take a break if there has been an intense period of trying and a baby is starting to show aversion. It can be wise just to drop the idea for a few days and have a fresh start later on. Most resources on paced bottle-feeding discuss the baby sitting in an upright position. However, there is sometimes a suggestion that a young baby may prefer a side-lying position (Pearson-Glaze 2022).

If a baby continues to refuse a bottle, we start to experiment with the variables. They may prefer a different temperature, location or person to hold the bottle. They may respond more positively when they are hungrier or *not* hungrier. They may accept a bottle when they are sleepy, such as during a 'dream feed'. They may respond to a teat being dipped in milk, or a dribble from a syringe alongside the bottle.

Sometimes, it can be useful to use distraction techniques. When we bounce gently on a birthing ball or make a loud 'chicka chicka' noise, half the baby's brain is engaged with a 'What on earth are you doing?' thought and the other half may object less to the introduction of the bottle.

If all this still fails, families need to know that there are alternatives. Very young babies can cup feed and videos online demonstrate the technique where a baby is encouraged to do their impression of a little kitten lapping milk (Global Health Media 2016). Soft cups designed for feeding young babies can be bought online and some have lips or spouts, like an Indian *paladai* (a feeding vessel which has been used for centuries). For young babies, finger feeding using a feeding tube might also work. A baby will need to be reclined, but not fully supine as that might increase the risk of aspiration. The caregiver can encourage the baby to maintain eye contact. They might talk and reassure as they insert the pad of their clean finger against the roof of the baby's mouth. A feeding tube can be placed against the roof of the baby's mouth, or in the corner of their mouth, and as the baby creates a vacuum, milk will be drawn through the tube. A bottle that is held higher up will elicit a faster flow. As breastfeeding professionals, we need to bear in mind that this will not be the manufacturer's intended use of the feeding tube, and we will bear the risk for that.

As a baby gets older, and especially if a family is transitioning from breastfeeding after six months, moving straight to cups and skipping the bottle stage may be preferable. They may choose to use a larger open cup. Some brands are made on a natural slant to make self-feeding easier and require less tip for the milk to reach the baby. A free-flow sippy cup may also be an option. Some open cups have a mushroom-shaped insert which minimizes spills. A straw cup is also an option, especially from around nine months. Some brands allow you to squeeze a little up into the straw to encourage drinking.

Of course, the loss of breastfeeding is also the loss of one of the best cuddles in the world. A baby feeding from a cup needs cuddles, and we must be careful that self-feeding is not an early expectation. When we talk about a baby under 12 months transitioning from breastfeeding, it is easy to get wrapped up in dropping breastfeeds and discussions of milk volume, but we must never lose sight of the fact that breastfeeding was about connection and an exchange of love and physical affection too. It was about oxytocin. We still want that oxytocin creation to happen. We are not simply losing breastfeeding but adding in a new method of feeding *and* lots of opportunities for physical affection. Bottle-feeding can happen skin-to-skin. A parent and a baby can bathe together and co-sleep, and when bottle-feeding does happen, it is a communication exchange, as well as an exchange of milk.

There is one final consideration when we discuss weaning under 12 months. Sometimes we will meet a parent who describes their child as 'self-weaning' under 12 months. It might be accompanied by a sense of relief and completion, or feelings of distress. As IBCLC Kelly Bonyata says,

> When a mother says that her baby self-weaned before a year, there is a chance that she interpreted a normal developmental stage (perhaps combined with her own wishes) as baby's wish to wean. Low milk supply can also play a part. (Bonyata 2022)

What we may be seeing is a baby who is developing a preference for the flow of a bottle. It may also be a child experiencing a nursing strike (which is particularly common around nine to ten months). A key question is whether the 'weaning' is abrupt because child-led weaning is very unlikely to happen. However, I would question the concept that breastfeeding professionals and volunteers are officially the gatekeepers of the definition of child-led weaning. I believe it is possible for a 10- or 11-month-old baby to not have an emotional relationship with breastfeeding and for their enthusiasm to fade away. They may have lost interest in breastfeeding to provide comfort or to aid sleep, and once the world becomes more exciting and they are more mobile, breastfeeding has less value. The key question is how the parent feels about the situation and whether they need our support. As a breastfeeding supporter, helping a distressed parent resolve a nursing strike will be an area you are already familiar with.

We often use the term 'nursing strike' to describe the experience of a nursling abruptly ending breastfeeding, although the word 'strike' is perhaps unhelpful as it implies this is a conscious decision on the part of the nursling, and the parent is presumably meant to meet some demands and then the strike will be over. The trouble is that they usually don't know what the motivation is and what the demands are. It's like when workers go on strike and refuse to tell their employer what their issues are. They are picketing with signs that don't have any words written on them. They are angry at meetings where no words are spoken. A baby or toddler who previously breastfed happily and enthusiastically seems to have had a switch flipped and the breast has suddenly become their least favourite place to be. For parents, it can be incredibly confusing and distressing. Parents can feel as though they are expected to switch into Sherlock Holmes mode at a time when they feel rejected and upset.

First, the parent needs to give themself some space to acknowledge that this *hurts*. Not so much physically, although they do have to be careful not to get engorged, as that might mean supply reduction and blocked ducts. This hurts emotionally. Feeding their child has been happening for several months and it is part of who they are. They may feel they are part of a community online and in real life, and that appears to have changed overnight. Their breastfeeding relationship with their child may be the core of how they connect with them. It's far more than milk. It's how they soothe them, help them get to sleep (perhaps multiple times a night) and how they check in when the world seems big and scary (for either member of the dyad). That feeling of loss can be significant.

This is not simply about rejection. Their child seems to be a different person. They are no longer their partner in the breastfeeding relationship. They might feel like an adversary. They have spent months developing an understanding of their child. They feel they *know* them. Now their child feels like a complete mystery. They are rejecting milk, but it can feel like their understanding of their child has been rocked and they are rejecting *them*. For the first time, this person feels like a stranger. The act of trying to convince them to restart can feel 'off'. Everything they have read says this is a strike and they are very likely to restart breastfeeding at this age. But the parents also absorbed deep in their soul that the ideal is 'child-led' and 'responsive' feeding. So, to try to trick them to do something their body seems to be rejecting runs counter to that instinct.

What might be going on? We're not talking about an older toddler who has been winding down for a while: perhaps one or two feeds a day for ages. They may have skipped the odd day. Breastfeeding is not at the heart of their lives and they are clearly on the home stretch. We're talking about a keen breastfeeder, who fed multiple times a day and has gone from several feeds to nothing overnight. Sometimes the cause is obvious. They might have sores in their mouth from 'hand, foot and mouth disease', a very common early childhood virus. They might have chicken pox or a mouth injury or oral thrush. They might be struggling with a tough few days of teething. They might have a cold and be blocked up and it's a struggle to breathe when breastfeeding. If there has been a recent virus, it can be worth visiting the family doctor to rule out a lingering ear infection which can be the underlying cause of breast refusal.

It might be that they are reacting to a particular phase in a parent's menstrual cycle. It's not a universal experience, but sometimes fussiness can correspond to an imminent period, particularly the first one. It might also be that the parent is in the early stages of an unknown (or known) pregnancy. During pregnancy, some nurslings are completely unaffected and happy to continue throughout. Others are more sensitive to early hormonal changes and may even be affected in the first few weeks. They may also be less keen to feed when colostrum arrives during the second trimester (which will happen even if a parent is currently breastfeeding an older child). Lactose levels will drop which means less sweetness and some older verbal children even describe milk as tasting more like crisps (not a bad thing for everyone).

Pregnancy may also mean a supply drop, again in the first few weeks for some. About two-thirds of pregnancies do seem to mean a reduction in milk supply. For some nurslings, that's a deal-breaker. It might mean that some older children stop breastfeeding entirely. For some, it might mean more fussiness. Some may pause feeding for even a few weeks and then be keen to resume again after birth.

If you look online for other causes of a nursing strike, you might see a discussion of the baby reacting to a different perfume, soap or deodorant. I'm not convinced by this one as I've seen toddlers breastfeeding in a bath with a bath bomb while holding a piece of cheese. I'm not sure that devoting hours to hunting for a new scent in the home is the best use of a parent's time, but it may help them feel as though they are taking action and trying to control a situation where they feel helpless.

You may see discussion of a nursling reacting to visitors or a change in circumstances or increased stress. However, some nurslings will react to all those things by breastfeeding *more*. I'm a bit concerned when I see articles discussing how the trigger might have been a parent's return to work or the fact they have moved house or had a bereavement. It's not as though a parent can undo those things and we may get into a self-fulfilling prophecy where a parent's anxiety about an imminent nursing strike could project onto the nursling. But perhaps knowing that it might happen may mean they are at least prepared for the possibility.

Sometimes a biting incident may have been the trigger. This is an age where a child may experiment with teeth at the breast, or adjust their latch as new teeth come in. If a parent gets a shock and yelps loudly when a child unexpectedly bites, this may cause the child to be wary of coming back to the breast. This can feel awful because a parent can see how their reaction has freaked the child out and they can feel entirely responsible, so some self-forgiveness is needed. Truthfully, a parent may never know the cause. In many cases, the cause is not obvious. At a time when a parent is already feeling low, and they are missing out on the usual oxytocin too, they can feel worse by focusing on the necessity of being Sherlock Holmes. It might be more positive to focus on the solutions.

Whatever the cause, the list of suggestions for parents is fairly universal:

- Use some acting skills. This means keeping the pressure off and don't make it obvious that the parent is distressed and desperate. The parent is nonchalantly lying on the sofa with their t-shirt off watching their child's favourite TV programme and if the child happens to toddle across and wants to breastfeed, that's great. The parent isn't forcing the child towards them or pleading or bribing. The breast mustn't become a battleground.

- Keep parent and nursling close. They can bathe together, use a sling and lie together. The parent's body and breast are still their child's friend and the place where they are safe and secure. We don't want the only time the child hears the click of a nursing bra to be, 'Uh oh, this is the bit where she tries to get me to breastfeed again.' The breast is just *there*. It's no big thing.

- Use of sleepy time. This is often the key. Many times, a strike ends because of acceptance of a breastfeed when a child is falling asleep, transitioning between sleep cycles or very sleepy. This is when co-sleeping can be useful because a parent is part of the furniture, and they can experiment with offering at different times in their sleep cycle.

- Use of 'distracted brain' time. When a child is sleepy, and most of their brain is busy focusing on something else, we can offer when they are only half-noticing. We can also exploit the 'half-noticing' when they are awake. There is a video of lactation consultant Edith Kernerman working with a baby who was reluctant to feed. You can read some of Edith Kernerman's thoughts on breast refusal online (Kernerman 2011). She had the mother bouncing on a birthing ball (or was it moving on an office chair?) while loudly saying, 'chicka chicka chicka'. The baby had this expression of wonder, like they were thinking, '*What* are you doing?' and was so distracted they didn't seem to mind being asked to latch on. Latching might happen when they are in a sling and the parent is walking outside, singing, talking and swaying.

- Sometimes the complete opposite might also work. A parent can go into a distraction-free room. They could even black out a room and see what happens.

- If the child does have a sore mouth, oral gel might help, and a parent can talk to their family doctor about options. Sometimes a breastmilk ice-lolly can bring relief and it's also a way to get milk into them.

- A parent will need to think about how the baby will be fed. Obviously, this depends a lot on how old they are and how they are getting on with solids. A parent should be encouraged to not automatically think, 'My child is X months old so their 24-hour intake of milk must be Z ml. Therefore, I must pump and give non-human milk if necessary, but it must be Z ml total in 24 hours.' We don't want a baby to be dehydrated but a little bit of hunger may be a motivation, and if a parent is giving vast amounts of milk, you may be removing that motivation. If they are giving milk using a bottle, they may also be meeting their need to suck. Some suggest offering milk via a cup, spoon or syringe while a parent is trying to encourage them back to the breast. If the nursling is happy to suck on a finger, you might be able to finger feed with a feeding tube.
- A parent needs to protect their supply. If their child is older, their supply will be less vulnerable than it was in the early weeks. However, production still operates on a supply-and-demand basis. Over time, if milk isn't removed, supply is likely to decrease. Expressing approximately when the nursling might have fed is probably sensible. If supply was to decrease further, a slower flow might mean that they are less keen at the breast. Sometimes slow flow was partly the reason behind the initial reluctance so some work on increasing supply might be useful. Occasionally, fast flow is the problem, and a strike occurs if a nursling just can't face coping with being overwhelmed.
- Use expressed milk as part of the strategy at the breast. Trickle milk over the nipple. Let the child suck milk off a finger. Or express milk just before an attempt to help the flow to get started.
- Is anyone else around to model breastfeeding? There's an unverifiable story of a gorilla learning to breastfeed by watching a human mother (Breastfeed LA 2019). A more recent story involved an orangutan in Virginia learning from watching a zookeeper (Saunt 2023). A parent could visit a group where breastfeeding will be happening or get a breastfeeding toddler to visit, or pretend to breastfeed a toy or another object.

- Sometimes it's wise to stop trying for a little while. It can take the pressure off to have a break, even for a couple of days, and then try again.
- A parent may be surrounded by people who don't quite get what the problem is, who may feel the parent has already been breastfeeding for quite long enough, and even see this as an opportunity. An early priority would be for a parent to communicate why this matters and what they need from their support network. Failing that, they may want to reach out to online breastfeeding support communities or local peer support.
- If nipple shields or bottles are already part of a dyad's life, they may be a tool to help bring a baby back to the breast. This might mean loading a nipple shield with milk, so they immediately get a mouthful, or starting with a bottle and then quickly switching to the breast. They can also bottle feed while skin-to-skin.

There is not a standard length of time for a nursing strike, and no one can tell you exactly when it might end. I have personally worked with mothers who experienced a strike for two or three weeks and their toddler did resume. I have also worked with mothers who just struggled for 24 hours. I've heard of nursing strikes that go on even longer than three weeks, although that is unusual. Sometimes an older child may stick with breastfeeding only at night or when they are sleepy, for a while.

When does a parent 'give up' trying? No one can answer that question for someone else. If we say that sometimes nursing strikes last for three weeks, that does not mean that a parent is then required by law to live in a state of desperation for three weeks and continue to work hard to resume breastfeeding. What about if you have an 11-month-old who was feeding twice a day and now they aren't interested? They are calm. There's nothing else going on, but they aren't interested. Is that a nursing strike? Or maybe it's self-weaning? Perhaps those previous two feeds corresponded with patterns in the daily routine and those patterns have changed and they are not bothered about the loss of breastfeeding. Is that a strike? There is no 'International Committee of Self-Weaning' that will hear a dyad's history and decree whether or not a child's story fits the criteria. Truthfully, self-weaning at 11 months is unusual but we have described a toddler who naturally drifted away from breastfeeding. That's not the same as a toddler who is a 'boob monster', feeding four to eight times a day, who suddenly overnight behaves very differently.

Most nurslings in the 8–12 months age range *will* restart breast-feeding. We wouldn't be here as a species if nursing strikes meant the end of breastfeeding for children this young. However, a parent is an expert on their child. If a parent has a younger child who has moved away from breastfeeding, and they feel at peace with the idea that this decision was child-led, our role is going to be acceptance rather than submit a report to that 'International Committee of Self-Weaning'.

Lizzie describes her daughter's sudden weaning at ten months:

One evening my nursling just decided she did not want boobie/ breastmilk anymore; she had one little suck and then refused. The next day she wouldn't even latch. I kept casually offering for about two weeks but was pushed away and refused every time. I had returned to work about six weeks prior to this; days I was working she would have oat milk from a straw cup with her dad. I don't know if it was a preference for the oat milk or the ease of drinking from a straw, but this was what she wanted. I felt really quite low at the time; I was not at all prepared for stopping so suddenly – literally it was out of the blue – we didn't have that last 'moment' where I knew it would be the last time I nursed her. I also felt feelings of guilt for having returned to work and so I was not with her 24/7 anymore, and wondered if this is why she didn't find comfort at the breast anymore. Later then came the relief – maybe once my hormones had levelled out and I came to terms with the sudden change, I actually felt happy that it had been my daughter's decision to stop, rather than mine, and relieved that I could stop expressing and anyone could now feed her without any trouble at all.
(*Lizzie*)

You can see how, despite Lizzie's initial distress, the abrupt nursing strike eventually felt like a form of self-weaning that did bring Lizzie peace. It would be hard to make a case for this not being 'self-weaning', nor should that be the call of the breastfeeding supporter. What do you imagine Lizzie's daughter would perceive it as?

I have occasionally spoken to parents who were advised, by family members and sometimes health professionals, to wean at a year or soon after, because it will be 'easier'. These are the moments as a breastfeeding professional where you take a deep breath and attempt to remain professional. The word 'easier' seems to be referring to the concept that there is less of a battle or less protest from a child. Let's not imagine that a pre-verbal child is still not feeling an impact, even if they are unable to express those feelings and have them understood by the parent. The 'easiest' time to wean a child is the hour before they were due to self-wean anyway. The preferable time to wean a child is when the parent wants to end breastfeeding. By perpetuating the myth that a younger child is 'easier', we are depriving families of the indisputable physical and mental health benefits of breastfeeding when they may have happily continued for longer. A child who is older and able to communicate can collaborate in the process and that can be a gift. Every child is different and every relationship to the breast is different, and the 'professional', who I heard about recently, who advocates all parents wean before 18 months, because otherwise 'it gets harder', needs to meet some more 18-month-olds and better understand the concept of evidence-based practice. An infant who experiences the loss of breastfeeding needs empathic and sensitive parents who understand that this is only partially about a milk delivery system. Both members of the dyad need continued opportunities for skin-to-skin holding and physical contact. Whenever breastfeeding ends, the impact will be felt.

Chapter 6

Weaning in an Emergency

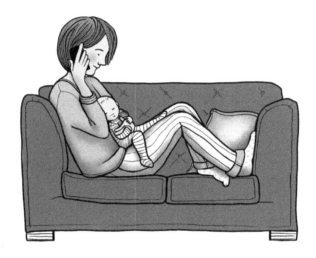

When weaning needs to be led by a parent, we usually suggest that gradual weaning is ideal. This gives breasts a chance to adjust and minimizes the risk of blocked ducts and mastitis and potentially gives both child and parent a chance to adjust emotionally. However, sometimes this may not be possible. The cause may be a parent's medical diagnosis; breast cancer, or the need to start another cancer treatment, could be the issue.

Dr Justice Reilly (Dr Justice Reilly – Breastfeeding Medicine: https://breastmed.co.uk/) is uniquely placed to support parents who may have to stop breastfeeding suddenly or navigate their breastfeeding journey alongside medical treatment. She is one of the few medical doctors in the UK who is also an IBCLC (International Board Certified

Lactation Consultant), and is in addition an NHS specialty breast doctor based in Glasgow, Scotland:

Q: What are some of the circumstances that lead to a parent having to end breastfeeding suddenly, when neither parent nor nursling might want to?

A: These situations are thankfully rare but can make a difficult situation even harder. Nursing parents who have to undergo chemotherapy or take radioactive iodine treatment will have to abstain from breastfeeding.

Q: Are there times when a parent is told they have to stop breast-feeding and that isn't necessarily the case?

A: Historically there have been many medications that people were told they couldn't take while breastfeeding. Thankfully we have much more research now and can prove most are safe. We also need to consider the impact of not breastfeeding on the physical and mental health of the pair. Unless the baby has free and easy access to donor human milk, it is likely the risks of not being breastfed are higher than any potential risk of medication exposure. We know now that even in cases of maternal HIV infection, babies can be breastfed so long as they are exclusively breastfed and there is lactation support to help avoid nipple trauma. This is because the infant gut lining functions normally and fights infection when exposed to a diet of only human milk, so there is little chance of transmission of HIV. It was previously thought this should only be the case in low-resource settings where bacteria in formula powder cannot be eliminated with boiling water; however we now have guidance to support breastfeeding for HIV-affected families in the UK too.

Q: If a mother is told she has to stop breastfeeding in order for a scan or test to be possible, is that always the case, and what sort of time frame are we looking at for a scan to be effective?

A: Most scans can be performed without interrupting breastfeeding.

For breast imaging, we can perform ultrasound, mammogram or MRI (magnetic resonance imaging) with gadolinium contrast. It is recommended that the person feeds or expresses their milk immediately before the scan to get clearer images. In the UK, our Royal College of Radiologist guidelines state that someone may opt to postpone imaging until they have stopped breastfeeding for at least three months. The problem is that we recommend breastfeeding to two years and beyond, and some people will still produce milk after that time, even when they have stopped feeding/pumping for three months. People who have a strong family history of breast cancer, have BRCA (BReast CAncer) genes or have come through breast cancer treatment themselves will understandably be anxious and not want to delay screening. Ultimately it is the patient's choice to go ahead or not, but some breast-team members do need reminded of this from time to time. I have also spoken to breast radiologists who have found that after breastfeeding for a year the breast tissue does not appear to be dense and difficult to interpret, but we need some proper research in this area.

Q: How do you navigate working alongside colleagues and professionals who may be less informed about breastfeeding?

A: I think most people are open to learning, but we have often formed such fixed beliefs depending on our culture, and professional and personal experiences. It can be confronting to have the management you previously advocated challenged. There is not much lactation education in the breast surgical curriculum and like many specialties, anecdotes get passed down from senior colleagues. Ultimately as clinicians, we are all here to serve the best interests of our patients and should be continuing our professional development throughout our careers. I have worked with some amazing colleagues who may have never breastfed themselves but are really open to learning more and advocating for families with a holistic approach. Not all breast-team members only care about cancer! The real problem is our overstretched services and not the staff themselves.

Q: What are the particular challenges of supporting a mother who has been diagnosed with breast cancer while breastfeeding?

A: Having a cancer diagnosis while breastfeeding can feel like a betrayal. We are taught that breastfeeding reduces breast cancer risk, and while that is true, the risk is never 0 per cent. We can't technically diagnose breast cancer until the biopsy sample has been reported by a pathologist, but we can usually tell if there is a high degree of suspicion, on the day, based on the mammogram and examination findings. Sometimes a well-meaning doctor will suggest weaning at that initial appointment, which may not be necessary at all, or it puts unnecessary pressure on someone at an already stressful time.

Q: If a parent asks for help to wean in a short period (in less than two weeks), what key things would you want them to understand?

A: Firstly, it may not be necessary. Younger babies tend to accept bottles easier, and older babies might be ready to move onto cups. It's the emotional connection that people often find the hardest though, when their baby is rooting and looking to breastfeed and their parental instinct is telling them to respond to that, but they feel they can't. Stopping suddenly even when it's desired often impacts maternal mental health and people should be made aware of that. Donor milk may also be available for some time, even if the baby is older, which can ease feelings of loss for the mother.

There are a few ways to approach emergency weaning. If their child is close to stopping anyway, two weeks may be easily achievable with distraction techniques during the day and cuddles from another caregiver at night. Some people will use that time to savour the last breastfeeds though, or hold onto dream feeds at night to relieve engorgement and ease anxiety symptoms. With breast cancer, usually, surgery comes before chemotherapy so there will be separations and bandages on the breast, and at that stage, the baby might be able to understand nursing isn't an option if both breasts are being removed (bilateral mastectomy). People can take medication to stop lactation (cabergoline in the UK) the day before surgery if they plan on stopping feeding completely. Or they might use that time to concentrate on feeding from the unaffected breast, so they unilaterally wean the breast that is going to be operated on. If that's the case, they may need the team to express milk from the unaffected breast during surgery to prevent mastitis.

Q: In your experience, how often do parents restart breastfeeding after treatment has finished?

A: It is more common to resume breastfeeding or relactate when the baby is younger; that's because their suckling reflexes are stronger, and it is easier to have them nurse directly after a break. It's also possible to have a friend or sister wet nurse to maintain the suckling skills. Some people do express their milk longer term and usually those are people who have breastfed an older sibling and recognize the importance of human milk feeding. There's not a huge focus on preserving breastfeeding throughout or after breast cancer treatment in the UK. Understandably the focus is on cancer outcomes and survival for medical teams. Pregnancy-associated breast cancer makes up only a few per cent of all breast cancers and, through my various volunteer roles, I'm made aware of five or six UK cases a year who want to explore all their lactation options after diagnosis. Only one or two of those will continue to feed after surgery, mostly because their hormone therapy is recommended for five years after surgery, and they know prior to surgery this isn't compatible with breastfeeding. I feel passionately that people should be allowed to explore all their options, make informed decisions and still feel they have a choice, especially in these difficult circumstances. Finding ways to honour their journey, like taking nursing pictures, writing a journal or commissioning milk jewellery can also help ease the transition.

(Reilly 2022)

This book discusses weaning so we are assuming lactation is already established. In some cases, cancer treatment will have been happening before pregnancy and during pregnancy. There are other questions around establishing breastfeeding and whether breastfeeding is possible (and for how long before treatment might be resumed) that will vary according to each situation.

Reilly mentions that medication to stop established lactation may sometimes be used. Bromocriptine and cabergoline are often cited as options around the world. These drugs work by inhibiting prolactin secretion. Prolactin is required for milk production, and endogenous dopamine inhibits prolactin release, so low doses of dopamine agonists like cabergoline and bromocriptine can be used to suppress prolactin production. Bromocriptine is now considered not to be a first choice as its side effects can be significant.

As the Canadian Paediatric Society states in the position statement on weaning:

Bromocriptine (Parlodel, Novartis Pharmaceuticals, Canada), a prolactin suppressant, is no longer licensed as a 'dry-up' medication. There have been reports of serious adverse drug reactions in the mother, such as seizures, strokes and even death, associated with its use. (Grueger, Canadian Paediatric Society and Community Paediatrics Committee 2013)

Cabergoline is considered a preferred option, though is not entirely benign:

Among a total of 757 women, 108 adverse events were observed in 96 women (14.2%). The most common adverse events were dizziness (35 of 757), headache (30 of 757), and nausea or vomiting (19 of 757). These events were described as short-lived, self-resolving and dose dependent. One pharmacovigilance study reported 29 'serious' events from a total of 175 events in 72 case reports, which included thromboembolic and neurologic events. Four case studies specifically addressed the psychiatric population, with one-half reporting psychiatric symptoms following administration of cabergoline. In conclusion, this systematic review demonstrates that adverse events were generally benign and tolerable following the administration of cabergoline. However, pharmacovigilance data reveal that vigilance is still needed given the occurrence of rare but serious events. (Harris *et al.* 2020)

Cabergoline is sometimes given for lactation suppression after the loss of a baby when ongoing lactation for milk donation is not desired. However, there are contraindications:

It should not be prescribed for women with pre-eclampsia or hypertension. Other contraindications include severe hepatic dysfunction, history of puerperal psychosis, cardiac valve disease, and pulmonary, pericardial and retroperitoneal fibrotic disorders. It should not be prescribed to women with sensitivity to ergot alkaloids, or women on antipsychotic medication. (University Hospitals of Leicester 2021, p.2)

If lactation already exists, doctors can prescribe cabergoline (250 micrograms) as an oral tablet every 12 hours for two days (total of four doses).

When lactation needs to end quickly, perhaps to aid greater visibility during a scan, you can see how a pharmaceutical option to speed up the process seems appealing. Chapter 4 also discusses the use of pseudoephedrine and some herbal options. However, speeding up the physical process of milk removal may not make the emotional impact of sudden weaning easier. In most weaning situations, someone wants to end breastfeeding. It will either be the nursling, in the case of child-led weaning, or the parent in the case of parent-led weaning. Now imagine the emotional maelstrom when neither party wants breastfeeding to end.

Parents who are embarking on medical treatment can often feel as though they are letting their child down, even though their logical brain knows this isn't fair. They can be worried by both the impact of this on their relationship and that they will be separated from their child. They can also be worried that there might be an ongoing struggle to care for their child if they feel unwell. Just when they are concerned about themself, they feel overwhelmed by apprehension about how changes might impact their nursling. To deprive them of breastfeeding at a time when the home is filled with an extra layer of emotions can feel especially cruel. A cancer diagnosis can come quickly for some families. One moment you are being investigated for what might be a lactation-related lump (which is surely more likely), and the next moment you might be considering surgery and possibly chemotherapy not long after.

Sometimes a parent might feel betrayed by breastfeeding, as Reilly touches on. Breastfeeding is touted as reducing the risk of breast cancer. Why didn't that work for them? They may even feel angry that lactation masked a problem and delayed a diagnosis and now may even be delaying treatment. If they meet a health professional who is frustrated that there is a complication of breastfeeding, that can feel even worse. If a health professional doesn't understand why ending breastfeeding might feel emotional, and the parent feels their challenge is being belittled, that also doesn't help.

Emergency weaning looks like an accelerated version of any weaning. We try to be as emotionally authentic as possible. For a young child, that may not mean explaining a cancer diagnosis in detail, but it might mean talking about the fact that milk is going away and it is going to be hard for everyone, but the parent is there to support them. It's not easy to start weaning unless a parent has an understanding of what breastfeeding means to their child. Is it their way of connecting when they feel isolated? Is it their tool when they feel overwhelmed or overstimulated? Is it their tool for calming down and preparing for sleep? Is it a request when they feel bored, hungry or thirsty?

If a child is older and verbal, they are a partner in a collaborative process. The need to wean is discussed explicitly. What suggestions do they have about how their needs could be met? With younger children, breastfeeding has often become a language of connection. The physical connection can be met with cuddles and also playful parenting, which is discussed in more detail in Chapter 7. If the request is coming from a desire for greater emotional connection, a parent can offer an alternative which gives the child their focus and attention. Previously, a child's request for a breastfeed was a way of asking for a parent's focus, meaning 'I want you to give me your time'.

What else could fill that role? It might be a request to read a book (so there's a new box of books available or books are displayed in a new way). It might be that there's a new tent with fairy lights and they can take you by the hand and ask you to join them. A child needs a new thing to ask for, that they can feel control over. We want them to feel empowered in other areas of their life. Can they choose what is for dinner? Would they like to leave the park now, or after one more thing? It is also all hands on deck with a network providing support. Explicit conversations can happen throughout the day, where other family members talk about how they get to sleep or a time when they had to say goodbye to something important and offer the nursling attention and support. This new normal needs to be established quickly and it needs teamwork.

All the preparation in the world won't prevent a child from feeling a sense of loss and confusion. A parent who is already in the middle of one of the most stressful times in their life will understandably want all that to go away. They might even be tempted to go away and leave another adult to care for their child. However, their child needs to know that the parent is there to support them, whatever they feel will be 'allowed' and validated. If a child feels sad and angry, that will be understood and empathized with. A child isn't praised for staying quiet and making it easy. Their natural reaction is supported and understood. Night time is likely to be especially hard, particularly if the child has relied on breastfeeding to get back to sleep between sleep cycles. It is a time when even a verbal child may be less interested in discussion and reasoning, and it is a time when a parent who is being stretched to their limits can feel very alone. It can be helpful to have a second adult offering support during these nights, not because they are going to take the lead away from the parent but to provide back-up if they want to step away. A second adult may also have an early start to take the child downstairs, to avoid a morning feed and to allow the parent to sleep a little longer after a tough night.

Sometimes a parent may choose to wean only on one breast. Milk production does operate independently, and it is possible to dry up one breast and allow production to continue on the other. It is worth pointing out, however, that the concept of 'drying up' is relative. Many parents report that months, and even years later, some milk may remain. The act of 'checking' may continue the milk production process in itself. Author Joanna Wolfarth, in her book *Milk: An Intimate History of Breastfeeding*, describes a moment more than a year after she last fed her 18-month-old son:

> As I lay submerged in the bathtub...it occurred to me to wonder if my body still possessed the power to make milk...I gingerly reached for my breast. I squeezed the soft flesh, gently at first and then more firmly, remembering those instructional videos. Thinking about your baby helps the milk flow, they said. So I conjured a vivid memory of my son's mouth latching onto my nipple and the rhythmic tug of his suck. And then, slowly, thick dark yellow liquid appeared, like custard through a sieve. I dabbed at it with my finger, which I then brought to my mouth to taste. For some reason, I expected it to taste sour, like curdled milk left to solidify in an old bottle. But it didn't. (Wolfarth 2023, p.242)

This is a normal experience after weaning. If, however, a mother notices changes to her breast after a while and lactation appears to be kick-starting without any obvious stimulation, we would signpost them to their GP for assessment.

A parent who is having radiotherapy to treat cancer in another part of their body may be able to continue breastfeeding. If a parent is having chemotherapy, they may choose to maintain their milk supply with expressing throughout their treatment, to resume breastfeeding after treatment is finished. This milk needs to be discarded but the process preserves the option to breastfeed later. In some cases, with lower-dose chemotherapy, it may even be possible to breastfeed between treatments.

If breastfeeding can be preserved, and a parent wants it to be, that should be respected. As La Leche League explains:

Experience has shown that weaning will not help a mother 'conserve her strength'. Breastfeeding is considerably more convenient, relaxing, and timesaving than bottle-feeding. It provides an emotional connection and intimacy that is nurturing to both mother and baby when they need it most. (La Leche League International 2022)

Sudden weaning might also be required when a parent's circumstances change for other reasons. It might be the case that a parent falls pregnant and has a high-risk pregnancy. Pregnancy and breastfeeding are ordinarily compatible, but in rare cases, a couple may be advised not to have sex to avoid oxytocin surges, and breastfeeding may also be considered inadvisable. Parents feel guilty without much provocation and sudden weaning is a time when parents will need to be particularly forgiving of themselves. It's important to celebrate the breastfeeding that has occurred. It has given the relationship between parent and child a strong foundation and this will help everyone cope with an abrupt weaning process.

Chapter 7

~~~~~

Weaning a Reluctant 'Boob Monster'

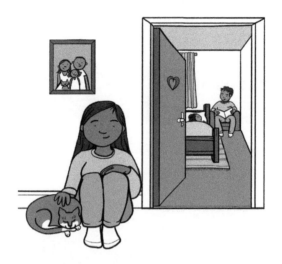

The term 'boob monster' or 'booby monster' describes a nursling who is an enthusiastic breastfeeding fan. These are not the three-year-olds who breastfeed around bedtime and maybe in the morning, but really could take it or leave it. These are the young children for whom self-weaning seems like a dot on a distant horizon. The parents of these children, who wish breastfeeding to end, are least serviced by concepts like, 'Don't offer, don't refuse': Don't refuse a child who breastfeeds five to eight times every night. Don't refuse a child who would remain latched on an entire night if that was an option. Don't refuse a child who would ask to breastfeed every single time a parent sits anywhere, in any building, at any time. These are the children for whom the breast seems like their best friend. Even the most loving parent can recognize that, and still be ready for breastfeeding to end. How do they even start? The process will be an individual one and it begins with a parent reflecting on what their process will need to be. The stages of parent-led weaning of an older toddler (and beyond) are as follows.

A *parent deciding to start*. They will reflect on their feelings about breastfeeding and their reasons for wanting to stop (see Chapter 2). They will give themself permission to dig deep and find motivations that are about them and what they want. They will allow themselves to prioritize their self-care and their own needs. Certainly, a nursling benefits from a happy parent. The last thing we want is for a nursling to sense that breastfeeding is happening reluctantly or miserably. However, weaning is not 'for the child' in that situation. It is for the parent – and that is OK.

A *parent needs to do a breastfeeding assessment*. Other words might be review/evaluation/observation. This is why there is no 'one size fits all' approach to weaning. What is this child's relationship to the breast? A parent will spend a minimum of a few days noticing their child's patterns. Are they more likely to ask at a particular time of day? Or when their parent is engaged in a certain activity? Are they hungry for food or hungry for connection?

A *parent needs to decide who their team will be*. Do they need to reach out to a breastfeeding support professional? Do they have a friend who can act as a mentor? How will friends and family be there for them? How much can the child themself be part of the collaborative and decision-making process?

A decision needs to be made on *how much a parent will communicate with their child* about what is to come. What language will they use? How will a parent answer the simple question, 'Why do we have to stop having booby milk?' How does a parent even introduce the subject? Can other carers use the same language?

It's necessary to reflect on *what a child will need to replace breastfeeding*. The act of weaning is not simply the act of removing breastfeeding. Many new things often need to be added. Some parents will learn to parent in different ways. A child will need a new language to replace the dialogue of breastfeeding, and may need a new language of nutrition and new strategies for physical contact and affection. They may need new ways to ask for help in emotional co-regulation. They may need a new language that helps them feel empowered and in control of their world. They may need a new language of sleep and getting to sleep.

Alongside these new languages and opportunities, *breastfeeding becomes more restricted and boundaries are put in place*. When there is an understandable emotional reaction, those *feelings are validated and supported*. There is space for sadness and anger. *Evaluation and reflection continue to happen* along the way.

Let's explore these stages in more detail. Chapter 2 discusses making the decision, so let's start with the breastfeeding assessment. With an older, verbal child, this can be a process that they are very much involved in. In the moment when a breastfeed is requested, what is a child's trigger? For some children, asking for a breastfeed is an easy substitute for the hassle of accessing a different drink – especially at night. It might actually be thirst. It could be that the issue is hunger. A parent might notice that a breast is requested mid-afternoon between lunch and dinner.

Does a child often request the breast outside the home when they are looking to check in with a parent and feel safe? Imagine a well-attached toddler is connected to their parent by a metaphorical stretchy piece of elastic: they might go off and explore their world and the elastic extends. They might spend a chunk of time playing with other children or talking to a new adult at a play group. Then they remember that the elastic exists and want to fill up their 'mummy cup' reserves again. If a young child can't say, 'Give me a moment. I just need to decompress after that new social interaction' or, 'This room is loud and busy and I'm feeling overwhelmed,' they may ask for a feed. A parent might notice that they ask for a feed when they feel socially anxious at other times, for example, in a new environment or around someone new.

Breastfeeding may be the way that a child connects with a parent and asks for their focus. A small person might not be able to say, 'Hey, you've been on that phone long enough. I want you now. Look at me. Show me that I matter. I need to know that I am important to you.' Requesting a breastfeed is a shorthand way of saying, 'That's enough time focusing on that other person/activity now'. It is a way of saying, 'I need you'. It is the reconnection after separation. It might be that they want undivided attention when other siblings are around. Or in the morning, after several hours of sleep, they simply want to feel close to a parent and feel like they are the centre of a parent's world. Breast-feeding is also a way to feel physically close. It is a perfect cuddle. If a family doesn't regularly ask for cuddles, or have a vocabulary for doing so, the breastfeed will fit that gap. Connected to this is the feeling of empowerment it can give a nursling. The child wants a connection with the person they love most in the world. They ask and it happens. That must feel very special.

When a nursling asks for a breastfeed, they have control over their universe. A young child has direct control over very little. As Sarah Ockwell-Smith says in *ToddlerCalm*, 'If we really think about how much control a toddler has, not only over their parents but over every facet of their own life, it is actually minuscule' (Ockwell-Smith 2013, p.93). Breastfeeding was something they could request and when the request was met, that felt empowering. They were able to stop a parent in their tracks.

Breastfeeding might also be what they do when they are bored. That might be a hard thing to hear for parents who are expected to be stimulating their child's growing brain to an expert degree, but sometimes home life is boring, particularly when parents have to bal-ance childcare with other responsibilities around the home. During the lockdowns of the pandemic, toddler nursing went supersonic, and many parents reported that the level of requests increased signifi-cantly. One mother mentioned to me that she realized she was her son's 'biscuit tin' (Mooney 2021) and just as an adult grabs a snack when they are bored, her breast was an easy time-filler. A child who is used to a stimulating nursery environment three or four days a week is thrilled to be home with mum on day five, but also not used to a less structured play environment, and a breastfeed can simply be something to do.

It may be that breastfeeding is the tool a child uses to physically calm themselves. It is how they wind down when they are buzzing. It is also often used as a tool for sleep. It makes biological sense when you think that breastmilk contains hormones that aid sleep – for both the nursling and the parent. Nurslings of any age can enjoy breastfeeding as a way to transition to sleep, whether it is for a nap, at bedtime or after waking in the middle of the night. Breastfeeding might also be their decompressing tool when they feel overwhelmed at other times. They may be experiencing physical pain or feeling unwell. They can feel afraid.

An older child may also be able to have some role in the observation phase. Are they ever able to verbalize their motivation for wanting to come to the breast? Are they 'heart hungry' (Flower 2019, p.155) – which might be broken down into 'cuddle hungry', 'time/attention hungry' and 'calm hungry'? Or 'tummy hungry' or thirsty? The process of encouraging a child to reflect on their motivation for coming to the breast can start long before the weaning process.

Once a parent has spent some time observing and reflecting on their child's relationship with the breast, they will have a better understanding of what gaps will later need to be filled. They can consider how they can give their child a new language. It might be a new language of sleep, empowerment, connection and affection or new approaches to nutrition or boredom.

Who will a parent's team be? This is going to be hard to do entirely alone. A parent will need to be prepared for feelings of guilt to bubble to the surface. It is also helpful to talk through strategies and be able to reflect on how things are going and whether some adapting is needed. It may be that a friend can fulfil this role or a partner. Some parents have the option of family members, although this is not always the case as some family members may not even be aware that they are still breastfeeding. It may be that support can be found in an online space, or by buddying up with someone else going through the same experience, even if there has never been a real-life meeting. Peer support can work brilliantly during the weaning process. The pandemic opened many professionals up to the possibilities of online support groups, and this works particularly well with weaning, as the chances of having half a dozen parents weaning older children in the same local area are small. Parents weaning older children have often returned to work, and an online group allows meetings during lunch hour or when working from home. We will discuss ways that professionals can support parents more in Chapter 12.

The nursling is part of the team. At the moment, breastfeeding is being used to solve issues and fill gaps. Weaning is not a simple case of removing breastfeeding. New approaches are going to be added and that can take some thinking about. Ideally, both parties are going to work in collaboration to find a solution. Weaning is not a battle of parent versus nursling. It is trying to find a new world with compassion that meets the needs of everyone. A lot is going to depend on the age of the child, but a child who is verbal and can comprehend what a parent is saying can be a partner in the process. A parent might start with conversations in daily life that explain that milkies don't last forever. These conversations can happen long before they are personalized to say, 'One day, *you* will not have mummy milk'. We want a child to understand that one day breastfeeding ends and that can be hard, but it ends for everyone eventually. In the park, a parent might point out an older child on a skateboard, 'I wonder how old he is. I think he's about ten. I wonder how old he was when he stopped having mummy milk and how he felt about that?' A parent might talk about people in the supermarket, characters in the background of picture books or television friends. Does Peppa Pig still have mummy milk? It is never discussed so we assume not. I wonder how old she was when she stopped. How does she get to sleep now? What does she do when she wants to feel close to Mummy Pig?

Role play with cuddly toys (or even not-so-cuddly toys) can also be useful: here is mummy teddy and baby teddy. Baby teddy is having milk at bedtime and in the morning and sometimes he asks during the day too. Mummy teddy says that she will do cuddles in the day and read books, but milk is going away in the day now. How is baby teddy feeling? What can mummy teddy do to help baby teddy?

Reading picture books about weaning can also be an extension of this conversation. For many young children, reading a book is a time when they are most likely to focus, and repetition is ideal to embed new concepts. There are many picture books about ending breastfeeding; however, the quality (particularly in the illustrations and printing) can vary enormously. Print quality can be lower for self-published books. It seems as though many commercial publishers have yet to recognize the significance of this market. I always recommend a printed copy of a book rather than an ebook. The illustrations can sometimes be used as a starting point for a conversation.

A Time To Wean by Marlene Susan, illustrated by Hayley Lowe (Susan 2018), is a book for the early stages of the conversation. It doesn't end with a child being 'done', and is a gentle introduction to the concept that one day Mummy's milk finishes, just as it does for many animals.

Some options focus on night weaning. A popular book is *Nursies When the Sun Shines*, written by Katherine Havener and illustrated by Sara Burrier (Havener 2013). The concept is simple: 'Baby goes to sleep, Mommy goes to sleep and nursies go to sleep'. When it's dark outside, no nursies, and when the sun 'beams through that window' it is full steam ahead. However, depending on where you live on the planet, the sun may not behave accordingly. Some parents make the book work by using a night light that indicates sun and moon symbols to denote wake-up time. *Milkies in the Morning* (Saleem 2014) is a similar concept. The picture shows a child who is clearly older, and there is a page which shows her distressed and struggling. It's valuable to have some acknowledgement that this process might not be easy. In *Sally Weans from Night Nursing* (Mitchell 2013), there is also space for Sally to feel sad and angry. The idea is that now both Mummy and Sally get a more rested night so they have more energy to do things the next day. Truthfully, Sally was probably getting a good night's sleep with some support transitioning between sleep cycles, but the concept may support some families' narratives.

There are some books that I would describe as emotionally heavier. It's always wise that a parent reads the book alone for the first time, and it is particularly the case with the following ones. *Loving Comfort* is written by Julie Dillemuth and illustrated by Vicky Pratt. In the book, Jack is getting older and sometimes forgets to ask for a feed. Night weaning happens with a maternal nudge and some tears and the end to his breastfeeding is presented as largely self-weaning with some chats to steer him in that direction:

> Mama talked with Jack lots of times about how weaning happens – that he was nursing less and less often, and soon he wouldn't drink Mama's milk at all. He was no longer a baby. He was a toddler and growing bigger and stronger every day. Sometimes this was okay with Jack. Sometimes, it was not. (Dillemuth 2017, p.20)

In *My Milk Will Go, Our Love Will Grow* by Jessica Elder, illustrated by Sheila Fein (Elder 2020), milk is 'going away' rather than through anyone's choice – 'My body can't make more' – and both mother and child have feelings about that and there is space for sadness. *Booby Moon* by Yvette Reid, illustrated by Camilo Zepeda, is becoming a very popular choice (Reid 2021). The moon sent booby milk when the child was a baby. As they get older, 'booby stays asleep at night'. The night before a birthday, the family releases a balloon and says thank you to the moon and booby milk flies away. This then means that future babies will have their booby milk. Again, there is space for grief and difficult feelings. The book contains some advice to check the weather and lunar calendar on a key night to make sure that the moon is visible, and the key day doesn't have to coincide strictly with a birthday. It's certainly a clear message (and it's possible to follow the theme without balloon littering). There isn't a focus on why breastfeeding ends, other than future babies might need it, and for older children, there might need to be some additional conversation. However, it's a nice concept to tie things up with the moon and create a rite of passage, and it's struck a chord with a lot of families. See Chapter 9 for a discussion of *Booby Moon with Two*, which focuses on weaning a toddler who is tandem nursing.

Some books focus on 'you are getting bigger now'. *Bye-Bye Nah-Nahs* (Rice 2017) is light on the text and doesn't mess around: 'You've grown bigger, baby, haven't you? Time to say, "Bye-bye nah-nahs!"'; it is available in some other languages too. *Boobies Go Bye-Bye: A Weaning Story* by Nikki Osei-Barrett and Cyana Riley, illustrated by DG (Osei-Barrett and Riley 2021), presents an abrupt weaning journey, which will be a choice that some families want or need to make. Mama decides there is one last feed and the next day there are plasters on her nipples. Faye is told that 'Mama's boobies are broken'. Faye is given support for her big feelings. In the beautifully designed *A Big Change for Seb* by Emily Hardwicke, illustrated by Lucie Cooke (Hardwicke 2021), Seb isn't quite big enough to be allowed to go on the tunnel slide. Mummy explains that milk isn't going to happen outside the home any more (a common step, rarely represented in picture books). He gradually focuses on other things and forgets that he wanted milk. He eventually gets to go down the rocket slide and feels a sense of achievement alongside the love and support from his family.

Bye-Bye Mommy's Milk by Melody De Visscher, who is a certified breastfeeding counsellor (De Visscher 2020), could be described as a workbook for parents and child. There are places to insert drawings and pictures to represent an individual journey, and a practical section for parents. *Goodbye Mummy's Milk,* by Mariapaola Weeks, also has some space for family members to record their thoughts and provide a drawing (Weeks 2022). I should declare that I get a mention on her support and information page. Unusually, this book gives space for Mummy to have some negative emotions around breastfeeding. There is a reason why breastfeeding is going away – it's not working for Mummy anymore. That is presented honestly and openly: 'Mummy pleads, "Stop twiddling! Try the other side!" Even though I try my best, my mummy wants to hide. Mummy growls, "I'm tired. I can't breastfeed like this forever"'. Weeks is a health visitor and paediatric nurse so perhaps that means she is more brave and confident about expressing the feelings of a parent who is struggling and getting ready for ending breastfeeding.

Parents may like to go one step further and make their own weaning book. Using online photo companies, it's possible to create individualized books using family photos with familiar phrases that give everyone a sense of ownership of the process. Young children often like to see photos of themselves, and you can include photos of their sleeping space, special toys and their favourite foods and activities.

Alongside reading picture books, eventually the time comes to put the theory into practice. A parent needs to explain to their child that one day milk will go away *for them*. They have had a special and beautiful experience (or language that feels more appropriate depending on the child's level of understanding). A parent might share pictures of early breastfeeding and share memories. They might talk about how they have loved breastfeeding and how special it is and how they will find it hard to say goodbye too. They can say that they know saying goodbye will be difficult, but they will be there to offer support and help them get through it.

This conversation doesn't just happen once but is sprinkled throughout some days at different times. It might happen at the park or during dinner. Ideally, it happens at times when emotions are steady to start with, and there is time to explore feelings that arise. A child as young as 18 months or 2 years old may not be able to articulate or even fully comprehend what is being said, but repetition may help, and it makes sense to try to offer some explanation rather than underestimate their level of understanding. A parent must reflect on how they will explain to their child *why* breastfeeding is going away. Some parents struggle with doing this authentically. You will see stories online of parents rubbing their nipples in unpleasant tasting foods or even chilli oil (ouch). You will see parents covering their nipples in bandages and saying that 'boobies are broken'. As breastfeeding supporters, it is important we don't judge a parent when they go down roads that feel uncomfortable, but this is a difficult decision to support. Parents do it because they don't want to face the emotional consequences of their child perceiving them as being the cause of their distress. They don't want their child to think that 'they' rejected it, but that the third party of 'boobies' is the culprit. I'm honestly not sure this kind of deception even achieves that goal. For nurslings, a parent *is* the boobies in many cases. Perhaps they did something to make this happen. They certainly don't seem to be doing something to fix it. Why isn't there a trip to the doctor for starters? Parents often take measures like this when they have struggled to find any alternative guidance.

Breastfeeding has been such an honest and beautiful connection. If a parent has breastfed their child for several years, it seems a shame to end it with something inauthentic and something they may later look back on with suspicion. Are we really protecting them? Or avoiding an opportunity for honesty and emotional learning? Is a parent choosing to lie rather than face an outpouring of emotion, specifically their child's understandable anger directed at them? As psychotherapist and doula Amanda Leon-Joyce (@thedoulamanda) reminds us, sometimes parents 'hide away from thinking about' the ending of breastfeeding (Leon-Joyce 2022). This can happen when parents ultimately believe they are doing something wrong. They believe it is wrong to *say* that they want breastfeeding to end, and they will look for a way to stop breastfeeding without expressing those true feelings.

> Weaning from breastfeeding is often the first grief, the first death, the first ending, the first break-up. As parents, it is very easy for the unworked-upon parts of ourselves to feel vulnerable and to push that vulnerability onto our children. We make them take the extra suffering that we are not able to take. We don't want to have a difficult conversation about an ending, so we push that difficult conversation away. In doing so, we increase what our children may need to carry. No one wants a parent to feel worse about an ending, but sometimes as the adults with the developed pre-frontal cortex, we have to take a minute to understand that this is a difficult situation, and the difficulty can't be removed. The difficulty can only be moved. The more of the uncomfortable stuff a parent takes, the less [a child] has to. (Leon-Joyce 2022)

Many parents fear saying something like the following words to their older nursling: 'I have loved breastfeeding you very much. It has been one of my favourite things to do in the whole world, but I'm ready to stop now. When you were a baby, you needed my milk because you couldn't eat any other food. Now you are older, breastfeeding is still really special to you, but I am ready to stop. My body is ready to stop making milk. I want to give you cuddles and play with you and sleep near you and help you when you feel sad, but we will need to learn new ways of being close that aren't breastfeeding. We are going to do this together.'

Many parents fear speaking so honestly. They want to say things like, 'Milk is going away because you are getting older' or 'I think we will both sleep better if we don't have milk at night'. Neither of those concepts makes sense to a child. Why is milk going away? They may feel they sleep better at night because they have milk. They don't want a parent to do this for them! If a parent can find a starting place that is truthful, they will be able to continue with that honest communication. Can they say, 'I am ready to stop'? Can they say, 'I know you are not ready to stop, and you might be angry that I am ready, but I'm going to help you say goodbye to milkies'?

Of course, a parent will need to adapt their language according to their child. A very lengthy explanation may not be absorbed. It may be preferable to stick to short phrases that can be repeated. A mother might feel more comfortable saying, 'Mummy's boobies are tired now. They have made milk for a long time. Mummy's boobies are going to stop making milk and we are going to say goodbye to booby.' A mother might switch between using the first person and the third person: 'My boobies are tired. Mummy's boobies are tired.' Young children may be in a phase of being attached to the use of the third person before they move onto using the first person, but we want them to understand a parent is talking about their feelings and their wishes.

A child who is pre-verbal or non-verbal can still understand before they can talk. Those children can still benefit from being sat down and having the situation explained. As Aletha Solter explains in her book *Tears and Tantrums: What To Do When Babies and Children Cry*,

> Children of all ages deserve to know exactly what to expect. It is therefore important to explain everything to them, no matter how young they are, because they understand language long before they can talk... It is then important to do as planned, because changes can be very upsetting to young children. (Solter 1998, p.92)

A nursling who is weaning reluctantly has every right to be angry. Just as a parent has a right to wean, a nursling has the right to be angry and disappointed. Any method that seeks to deflect that anger by pretending this decision has nothing to do with the parent's choice is depriving a nursling of emotions they are entitled to feel. In the long term, that may have an unhealthy impact on the honesty and communication within the relationship.

An older child might appreciate an official 'meeting'. It can even be recorded using something like Zoom meetings. Minutes can be taken, although we might not call them that. We can record the language they use and the suggestions they make. If they have ideas, they can be written down and referred back to later. It can feel empowering to them to know that their thoughts are being valued and it may be the very first time in their life that their words have been written down. You can refer back to the recording at a later date too and they may enjoy watching your meeting and remembering the discussion. They must understand the feelings they express are validated. Naomi Aldort reminds us that,

> Validating is its own result. It is not a method we use to control or change the course of a child's upset or behaviour. On the contrary, validation and focused listening are our way of making it safe for the child to express herself; it is our way of offering love and intimate friendship. The result of such validation is that the child feels safe to feel her feelings and to express herself fully. The most likely immediate outcome of validation is more crying, a tantrum or other forms of self-expression. (Aldort 2005, p.5)

There is a misunderstanding that validation is a tool we use to calm children down. When we say, 'I understand', we are hoping that this is enough to stop them from being upset, but things might be more painful initially. Psychologist Philippa Perry explains that validating your child's emotions is like 'steering into a skid when you're driving on ice' (Perry 2020, p.69). Eventually, you might regain control of the car, but it is going to be wobbly for a while.

An early decision a parent has to make is what their time frame will be. Child-led weaning takes place over months and often years. What is the time frame for parent-led weaning? There is an assumption that parent-led weaning should always be as gradual a process as possible, but again, there is no 'one size fits all'. A parent needs to make a decision based on the child's current feeding patterns and what their relationship is to the breast. A child who is entirely dependent on the breast for sleep and transitioning between sleep cycles throughout the night is likely to need a different approach than a child who feeds twice a day and has no sleep association. An older child may have an understanding of calendars and days and be able to be involved in the decision. In some cases, a very slow weaning process with a reluctant partner may not be the kindest thing, nor the gentlest. Some children just want the pre-discussion finished so they can begin the mourning process and move on. A very lengthy preparation process is not necessarily easier to cope with.

It is sometimes said that distraction is a valuable weaning tool. I have said it myself in the past. For much younger children, it can be useful as you seek to meet their needs in other ways as quickly and as effectively as possible. For older nurslings, distraction can be a form of betrayal. It means a parent is hoping to avoid upset, when in fact a true expression of feelings, and accepting and being alongside them, should be the goal. In *Raising Our Children, Raising Ourselves*, Naomi Aldort explains that:

> The message the child is internalizing when distracted is that something is wrong with having feelings... Therefore, when we notice a need to interrupt, fix, distract, or give advice, we can stop ourselves and explore the drive inside us. Avoidance is pretending not to notice a child's unwanted expression in hope that it will go away... The question always comes back to: Why do we want feelings and their expressions to go away?... Sadly, a child whose painful feelings are being avoided will indeed diminish or stop expressing herself and may even stop feeling them, becoming emotionally numb and hard to connect with. Or in the healthy child, she will escalate her communication by choosing provocative behaviours that may finally get our attention. In addition, when a parent uses avoidance, the child's needs will not be met, leading to more stress with its many difficult behavioural symptoms. (Aldort 2005, pp.114–115)

Distraction is often a self-protective device for the parent. It is natural to not want to imagine that a child is experiencing pain. If there is a way to avoid seeing distress or anger, that sounds like an ideal scenario. However, there is something inauthentic about attempting to wean from breastfeeding by stealth. Truthfully, it is an opportunity to explore a child's feelings and for a parent to demonstrate unconditional love.

Philippa Perry describes how distraction 'can be an insult to a child's intelligence':

> What message does distraction convey? Imagine you fall over and badly graze your knee; how would you feel if your partner, instead of being concerned or interested in the pain or the blood or the embarrassment, pointed out a squirrel or promised that you could play your favourite video game? (Perry 2020, p.79)

Distraction is attractive in the short term. It might feel like a handy short cut, but this may not be the best time for short cuts. Philippa Perry describes talking about a house key, rather than the breast:

> You can help them with their frustration rather than distracting them from it by saying, 'You are angry that I can't let you have the key. I can hear you are furious about it.' If you stay calm and contain your child's feelings, this is how they will learn to contain them. It might feel like a longer process than simply distracting them away from the key, but the time invested will help them internalize these skills for themselves. (Perry 2020, p.80)

Of course, it does depend on what a child's motivations for wanting the breast are. If a parent is simply their 'biscuit tin' as described earlier in this chapter, distraction and offering an alternative activity may seem more valid. Distraction may also be an option for a pre-verbal or non-verbal child with limited communication skills. But ideally, distraction should be on-topic and meet the underlying need. If the child is requesting connection and time with a parent, then offering a different loving-focused activity isn't a distraction so much as offering a new way to meet the same need. However, a child who is asking for connection, and is instead offered a screen and a snack, is not having that need met respectfully.

Offering a snack as a breast alternative is particularly problematic. Parents almost always have some reflecting to do around food and emotions. Many of us live in cultures where food is a 'language of love' – it is literally how we express love to others around us and it is often how we express love to ourselves. When we feel emotional and upset and overwhelmed, food, especially sweet food, is often a way we 'manage' those emotions, although actually we are repressing them. As Marion Rose expresses in *The Aware Parenting Podcast* (Rose and Stone 2019), feeling upset and feeling hungry can be confused by many of us. Adults may not be in tune with that difference themselves and may project that onto their children. Over time, children may not be in tune with their own ability to differentiate between what is hunger and what is feeling overwhelmed.

It is difficult because responsive breastfeeding emphasizes that breastfeeding is multi-purpose. It is not just delivering a meal. It is meeting emotional needs, aiding sleep and providing comfort. That is the point – something we have lost sight of in previous decades. However, at some point, we need to break that connection between food and comfort. That is not to say that using food for comfort is 'bad', something we should feel guilty about and something that we must always avoid for health reasons, but that we need to be aware of what is going on. If a child is saying they are hungry and asking for a breastfeed, can we offer to 'feed' their needs in another way? As adults, we all need to recognize what we are doing in our relationship with food to be able to help children to reflect on theirs.

If we see weaning from breastfeeding as a time to add new parenting tools and new languages, what can that look like in practice? A new language around thirst and nutrition is about providing opportunities. Does the child have a cup they can use independently that is within easy reach? Do they have a way to request snacks or to explain when they feel hungry? All they may be skilled to do in that situation is to ask for a breastfeed.

Giving a child a new language to ask for connection and affection is often at the heart of weaning from breastfeeding. When a child continues breastfeeding beyond infancy, the dialogue of requesting a breastfeed and having that need met can feel powerful and wonderful. The most important person in their lives is pausing and meeting their request. When they have that urge for parental love and a sign of affection, they have the tools to do that. If that tool is taken away and no alternative is given, the risk is that the child feels not only rejected but also disempowered and destabilized. That was the only way that they knew how to ask for a physical sign of love. It was the only way they knew how to say, 'Hey, I need you for a moment!'

The reconnection feed that happens when a child is reunited with their parent after a day of nursery and work is sometimes difficult to drop. That feed is a powerful moment for a child decompressing at the end of a long day and celebrating seeing the parent again. Parents often describe a child racing through a door and literally leaping on them. Breastfeeding plays the role of marking the transition back to being at home and under the care of the parent. This may need some thinking about. Some children will arrive home full of energy, and high-energy connective play and physical games may meet a need. Some are tired and are looking for a moment of peace. Activities like a hand massage or head and shoulder massage can be special, and the nursling might take the role of the facilitator and the expert. Doing yoga together and developing a new ritual, which might also include a need for a drink and snack, can be something both parties look forward to. Something fresh and new can bring a sense of excitement.

Dens are a great tool to give little people a sense of fun and excitement. It might be that when a child comes home, their parent is waiting in the den with something to 'show' them and something to share. Or if a child is home first the reconnection can start with a game of hide-and-seek. A parent can create a cuddle nook which may be a tent or a home-made den with cushions, bean bags and fairy lights. This isn't a place where breastfeeding happens but where reading and cuddling and other kinds of physical connection occur. It would be sensible to discuss in the morning what will happen at the reunion. Another caregiver can mention it and remind the child during the day. The parent might even be able to speak to them on the way home via a video call to prepare them for what is going to happen.

Before breastfeeding is stopped, it is sensible to already start to widen the child's vocabulary. How else can they achieve that goal of asking for connection and a parent's focus? If requesting a breastfeed is the *only* way a child can ask for physical affection or a parent's focus, that will need to be remedied. A parent can model by asking them for a hug. It may be sensible to develop a short phrase that is easy to say or a piece of personalized sign language. The parent asks the child for a hug, asks other friends and family and models the process. What else can a child request, giving them not only the opportunity for physical closeness and affection but also a feeling of empowerment and agency over their world?

It has been said that reading a book with a young child is a close substitute for breastfeeding. Does the parent have a set-up where the child can request a book? Is it time to move the books to an accessible level, display them in a more child-friendly way or put out a small selection for each day? We want the request to be fun. During the weaning process, it can be sensible to think of a few new activities, as novelty can have some appeal. Clapping games are short and focused and give a child an adult's complete attention. Games that involve touch and fun are valuable. If a little person is a fan of toy vehicles, a parent can take a large white sheet and create a personalized play mat with permanent pens. The parent then lies *under* the sheet to create the landscape, valleys and mountains with their body. As the vehicles are driven over them, the topography can shift, bringing lots of giggles. A parent under a sheet can't be anywhere else and a child feels empowered.

A breastfeeding parent may have been accustomed to using a breastfeed as a way to give attention. The child feeds and happily toddles off to play independently. If breastfeeding is going to end, there may need to be a new approach to play. It is *during* play itself that connection and attention happen.

Shelley Clarke is a parenting mentor based in Adelaide, Australia. Her resources include a course for parents called *21 Days of Play* (Clarke 2023b). She supports parents at lots of different stages, including the ending of breastfeeding. I asked her to talk about how she supports parents to end breastfeeding and how her philosophical approaches underpin that thinking.

Aware Parenting is a parenting approach founded by developmental psychologist Aletha Solter PhD (Solter 2022). Her six books detail the whole philosophy, which is a form of attachment parenting that deeply understands the needs of children, play, listening to feelings and recovering from stress and feeling overwhelmed. Hand in Hand Parenting is another approach that centres around the parent/child attachment and places connection at the heart of the relationship (Hand in Hand Parenting 2023). Both approaches are focused on attachment-style parenting with the added component of meeting everyone's needs, and both understand the importance of listening to feelings and are looking for the need underneath a child's behaviour.

When I was feeding my second child, I was breastfeeding all night long and feeling very exhausted. It felt like my only options were two extremes: ending suddenly and being 'tougher' or continuing in the situation where I feel exhausted and overriding my own needs. I found Aware Parenting and Hand in Hand Parenting, which aim to honour the needs of everyone in the family, and our family life drastically changed.

There are three core components of Aware Parenting:

1. Attachment-style parenting – attuning and meeting the needs of our children.
2. Non-punitive discipline – we are aiming to meet the need underneath our child's behaviour.
3. Recognizing our inbuilt mechanisms for recovering from stress and overwhelm – welcoming all feelings and listening to our children's tears.

Aware Parenting and Hand in Hand Parenting both understand the important process of crying and listening to children's feelings. When children have the space to express themselves, often difficult behaviours shift, including constant feeding (especially overnight), as was in my case. Crying is our body's inbuilt mechanism to recover from stress and feeling overwhelmed. When we have had a chance to release and express our feelings, we often feel relaxed and more comfortable in our bodies.

When my children were younger and upset, I would always jump in and quickly try to fix or stop their upset. I would want to fix everything and would often whip out the boob to feed and comfort my child. However, I learnt that often this was just suppressing their feelings. With my new understanding of listening to feelings, and crying being a helpful thing, I started to listen and hold space rather than just react and fix. One of the most powerful gifts we can give our children is being attuned and present to their needs. When we listen to our children's upset feelings and bring our attention, connection, and listen, it meets their deep need to be heard, seen and understood. We all want our children to feel heard and seen. When parents are ending the breastfeeding journey, we can reflect on how we feel when our children are feeling upset. Do we jump in and shush, pat or feed, often distracting our children from their feelings? Or can we be calm and present to what they are expressing? Aware Parenting often helps parents offer a loving 'No' to a child but then bring attention to and listen to the feelings underneath. It helped me to hold a 'loving limit' (a term coined by Marion Rose, PhD), where we are saying a loving 'No' to a behaviour but we are listening to the feelings underneath. Once I started to become comfortable holding space for my child's tears, they stopped requesting the boob for every upset and I was able to continue the weaning process.

Attachment play is another key aspect of Aware Parenting and is extremely helpful during weaning. I know breastfeeding is a source of comfort and connection that many mothers find hard to end, as they often feel as if they don't have anything else in their tool kit to support their child. This isn't true. You are the most important source of comfort to your child. You. Your presence. Your attention. Your love. Your ability to listen to their needs and play is a wonderful way to meet their need for connection and great to add in during this time. Play can be used for many different parts of parenting, but in the context of ending breastfeeding, there are several games that are wonderful to play. When we play with our children in this specific way, we are using laughter as another form of emotional release. Shifting the feelings from their bodies helps our children to feel relaxed and calm, and often sleep is greatly improved. There are a few key ideas when we are playing in this way:

1. Your child takes on the more powerful role (power-reversal games).
2. You take on the less powerful role (i.e. the fumbling, clumsy, weaker one).
3. Follow your child's giggles.

When you follow your child's giggles, they are laughing, which is helping to shift the underlying feelings. It is also helping with connection and closeness. Games such as rough housing are great, as are pillow fights; close snuggles on the bed and chasing games where your child tries to crawl or run away from you, but you can't quite catch them, are wonderful ways to build connection and release tension. Being there with your child and following your child's lead is the biggest thing you can do.

Every child will be different in how they want to play. A parent who is weaning can dedicate 10–15 minutes throughout the day, or whenever you can manage some one-on-one time: just you and your child and follow their lead. If they want to play a chasing game, hide under the blankets, jump on you or ride on your back while you pretend to be a funny animal, just follow their lead and see what brings the laughter. You are often meeting their need for connection without their needing to be on the boob. My children loved vigorous snuggles and a game called '100 kisses'. When they would ask for the boob and I wasn't willing to feed, I would offer a loving limit and say, 'Not right now, sweetheart', but then I might say in a playful, inviting tone, 'But would you like 100 kisses?' And I would start planting kisses on their hands and feet, while they were trying to crawl away laughing. This is how we can offer a loving limit in a warm and playful tone while offering connection and following their laughter.

Another type of play is 'symbolic play' which is where you might role play with your child. You might play out 'breastfeeding' with your child, where they play the more powerful role, and you might be the child or following how they want to play out the scenario. When we follow our children in symbolic play, we are helping them to process

their world. These new connections can be rich and deep
where previously you might have been in a pattern of j
them, these games can be nourishing and fun for everyor

When we are starting the weaning process, it is helpful to add
these games so we increase our tools and ways of connecting with our
child. It is important to give your child lots of information: what you
are planning on doing when you will feed and when you might play
instead. For example, you could say, 'We will have a bath, then a feed
and then we will play before bed', or 'Tonight sweetheart, we will feed
before bed and then when you first wake in the night, I will be there
to listen to your feelings'. When we have more ways of connecting we
can feed when it feels authentic and meaningful, and then use play
and laughter at other times to meet their needs.

When we are wanting to start the weaning process, it is important
to have a space to process our feelings about it. Having a friend or
Listening Partner to work, share and express your feelings with will
make a very big difference to how you feel throughout the weaning
process (see the Hand in Hand Parenting website for more information on Listening Partnerships). Once you have offloaded your feelings
then it is time to start noticing and looking to meet your child's needs.
Adding in more chances for play and connection during the day or
offering a loving 'No' and listening to the underlying tears can make
all the difference with weaning but also sleep. Night feeding due to
regular waking can be a huge source of exhaustion for parents; having
a 15–20-minute window of vigorous energetic play before bed can help
a child shift energy and tension from their body before settling down
to sleep. It may also be a time we need to offer a loving limit: instead
of 15 books to read before bed, we read two and then listen to any
crying or feelings our child might have sitting beneath the surface.
Often our children will sleep much better after a big cry before bed.
I want to be very clear: this is not controlled crying or leaving your
child alone when they are crying. This is holding space for them, for
their feelings and their tears, and creating a sense of safety for them
to express all of who they are. You are there with your child.

For me, the weaning process, which felt hard and full of trepidation, became a wonderful time of connection, laughter and knowing

that I was meeting my child's need to feel loved, heard, seen and understood. It became a time of fun, laughter and lots of snuggles and games, and I could feel the warmth between us. I hope that with these tools of play and listening to your child's feelings, that this time of weaning becomes one of deep connection for you too. (Clarke 2023a)

Alongside introducing a new language around connection and physical affection, other boundaries around breastfeeding are progressively being put in place. Breastfeeding might still happen in the day, but only in certain places, perhaps no longer on a particular chair or restricted to a less interesting and stimulating room. The feed is not being entirely denied but would the child really prefer a long feed in one particular place? Or the chance to play or read a book somewhere else? A parent might agree to do a feed for a short period and then offer a different activity that may be more appealing. There may not be a need for a straight 'no'. The child is offered a feed, but over time ideally, their motivation diminishes as other options seem more exciting. As well as restrictions around location, a parent might come to put restrictions at times of the day. Breastfeeding can become associated with particular slots in the day. If there is a request outside those times, a parent can say, 'Our next feed will be at X time'. There may be protesting and anger. Those feelings are validated but the boundary remains firm. Something else is offered which hopefully meets the need that breastfeeding was going to meet.

If an older child has been able to participate in the breastfeeding assessment and understand for themselves what their motivation for breastfeeding might be, the process is a learning experience for everyone. When they notice they feel like having a breastfeed, can they help you to understand what their needs are? Do they need Mummy's attention? Are they feeling like they need some peaceful time? Are they stuck for an idea of what to do? They may even be able to come up with some suggested activities or responses to each need. When parents are having these discussions with their children, they will be considering their 'zone of proximal development'. This is a concept from psychology and teaching. Parents will need to assess where their child's understanding is and appreciate that the learning that we are asking them to do is slightly beyond what they can do independently, and is something the child needs support to achieve. These are concepts that they can understand with adult guidance. Every child's zone of proximal development will be different according to their age, comprehension and language skills. There is not one universal way for all parents to have these conversations with their children.

This is an emotionally heightened time. A parent might lose patience or struggle after the tenth request for a breastfeed. Even the most empathic and loving parent has a day when they may struggle to hide their frustration. As Philippa Perry describes, older generations of parents often struggle to apologize and to admit when they have been wrong. If a parent speaks with frustration, they can acknowledge that and apologize and offer repair: 'Being sensitive to feelings and following rupture with repair is always better than stand-offs, battlegrounds and winning and losing' (Perry 2020, p.68). When a parent already feels guilt about the process of weaning, if they perceive themselves as putting a foot wrong, it can require some deep breaths and some self-forgiveness.

All through the process, a parent is not praising a child for acquiescing or a lack of protest. We are not rewarding or praising a child who represses emotion, nor do we praise a child who is cooperating with the weaning process – because what is that really praising? A parent might say, 'Thank you for helping me to find different things to do instead of breastfeeding', and that is different from saying, 'You are such a good boy for not getting angry' or 'You are such a good girl for crying less last night'.

Is there a time when a parent might choose to pause the process? Absolutely. The message that a child needs us to be consistent is not the same as saying that when a parent has started the weaning process, they have signed an iron-clad contract and they are stuck on the path until the end. If a parent has had a difficult four or five days of night weaning and putting boundaries in place, and the child seems to be getting more distressed rather than developing an acceptance of the new limits, a parent may want to take a step back and review. With a verbal child, it might be time to attempt more communication. Do they have any ideas about why this might be especially hard? As Hilary

Flower describes, 'Giving your child some choices as to the nature, the level, or the pattern of reductions can help him or her feel empowered and valued' (Flower 2019, p.151).

What is unlikely to be sensible is having one night off and then restarting trying to put boundaries in place. A confused child is an unsafe child. If a child's distress starts to feel too difficult, it is time to do some reflecting. How is the parent feeling about their motivation to wean? Are they experiencing a wobble in the face of their child's distress because they have realized that perhaps they aren't ready to end breastfeeding themself? Or do they still want to end breastfeeding, but their child's distress has triggered feelings of guilt, selfishness and shame? Most parents have had to work hard to overcome these feelings to even start weaning and have started the process already on shaky ground. Does their child need more time to accept new sleep associations that are replacing breastfeeding?

Aletha Solter has some valuable thoughts on our cultural attitudes to young children crying (Solter 1998). She says there has been a huge misunderstanding about children's tears and tantrums, going right back to the Middle Ages when children who cried were thought to be possessed by demons. Gradually attitudes shifted and it was no longer the children who were evil but the parents who had been too indulgent or not parented strictly enough. She says that 'adults often try to repress crying and children out of a misunderstanding of crying, and because it arouses their own unresolved stress and need to cry. This repression of crying is passed from one generation to the next' (Solter 1998, p.7).

Today, parents who have crying children may not be perceived as lacking in discipline, but we may imagine that they are doing something wrong. Do they lack empathy, attachment, understanding and communication? Surely, they can fix it. The judging looks in the supermarket certainly seem to indicate this. Truthfully, those judging looks are about the baggage and unresolved issues of the people giving them. When a child is distressed during the weaning process, it can feel particularly painful when a parent knows they could fix the situation in moments by simply offering the breast. This is when the initial motivations are so crucial and why weaning because of something like external pressure, rather than deeper personal commitment, can be problematic.

Solter suggests we rethink what is going on when a child is crying or having a tantrum. The process of crying provokes physiological changes that result in a positive state:

> Crying is a state of physiological arousal followed by deep relaxation. It is a very effective way to reduce tension and to lower one's blood pressure and heart rate... It can be considered a natural repair process that restores the body to a state of equilibrium. Crying is therefore not an unnecessary by-product of stress, but an important part of the stress relaxation cycle. When we cry as a response to emotional stress, we release energy, reduce tension, lower blood pressure and remove stress hormones and neurotransmitters from our body through tears, thereby restoring physiological balance homeostasis. (Solter 1998, pp.16-18)

We assume that successful weaning means a child peacefully acquiescing. Sometimes that will be true. A child understands and accepts your motivations and can collaborate to move forward and help you with the process. But tear-free weaning is not always the healthy option. Solter describes how different groups of children respond to another stressful event, admission into hospital:

> Psychologists have studied crying in children during the highly stressful experience of a long hospitalisation. Children who protested openly by crying and screaming at the beginning of their hospital stay showed better adjustment than the ones who were 'good' patients right from the start. The latter appeared to be calm and cooperative but were more likely to show signs of stress later on, such as regression to infantile motor behaviour, eating or sleeping difficulties and learning disorders. (Solter 1998, p.19)

Solter has some interesting ideas about the breastfeeding relationship. She suggests that babies who are allowed to cry naturally in loving arms and are not encouraged to repress their need to cry will wean themselves more peacefully than those who develop a pattern of using nursing to repress their emotional state (1998, p.67). I'm not sure I would go as far as to say that encouraging children to meet their emotional needs at the breast is problematic, but I do appreciate her encouraging us to reflect on our cultural instinct to repress a child crying and to believe that crying is some kind of parental failure. I can also appreciate the point that discouraging a child from crying sends a message that we are not loving them unconditionally despite their negative emotions. In the middle of a weaning process, accepting a child's anger and showing that you are there for them, even in those difficult moments in the middle of the night, is valuable. Too often, when a child cries during night weaning, a parent who has been conditioned to feel guilty about the process of parent-led weaning will wobble. Was this the right thing to do? Should they abandon the process entirely? Sometimes, the answer to that might be yes. But that decision is not being made for that night but rather for the next night and the next week and the next month.

This is the time for a parent to revisit their original motivations. Hilary Flower, who is referred to in more detail in Chapter 9, has a helpful discussion of red flags that parents need to pay attention to in their breastfeeding relationship:

> These are the signs that a breastfeeding relationship needs adjustment:
> You feel yourself withdrawing from your child.
> You hear an irritated tone in your voice when you say, 'Yes'.
> You feel you have no choice when it comes to nursing.
> You are prone to snapping at your child while breastfeeding.
> You are getting exasperated enough to consider weaning on the spot.
> (Flower 2019, p.149)

It may be that if night weaning feels particularly painful, more than it feels manageable, a parent decides not to go down the full road of weaning and pauses part way through the process. They may find that with some limits, red flags start to fade to pink or disappear entirely. However, some parents may still need to move forward, accept that crying is a child's human right and provide as much loving support as possible. If a parent recognizes one of these red flags, then it may not be sensible to abandon weaning because middle-of-the-night crying feels too selfish and unloving. This entire process is about balancing the needs of everyone. If a parent returns to feeling irritated and snappy during breastfeeding requests, no one wins and, arguably, the long-term damage will be far greater; weaning will need to be revisited, when parental reserves may be even lower.

Solter's discussion of something she calls 'the broken cookie phenomenon' is also interesting. Children may sometimes build up a need to cry, and in looking for that release they may fixate on something that appears relatively insignificant. In her example, a broken cookie becomes the focus of tears and tantrums. In reality, the cause may be something much deeper. In our context, a child may in fact be struggling with the end of breastfeeding; but appearing to be angry about something relatively small, or protesting about another choice a parent has made, is something they can express more easily (Solter 1998, p.85). During the weaning process, we can encourage parents to look out for anger being expressed in different ways. It may be that by accepting crying as a form of release and a natural expression of justified anger, a parent can cope a little longer with some unsettled nights.

Let's imagine that weaning has reached its natural conclusion and breastfeeding has ended. Some families consider a special event or celebration to mark the end of breastfeeding. IBCLC (International Board Certified Lactation Consultant) B.J. Woodstein describes the approach she took with her daughter:

> At six years old, my older daughter was nearing the end of her time breastfeeding. We were both sad about this period of our life together coming to a close, but she was feeding less and not getting much milk out when she did. Over some months, we discussed how it might feel to stop feeding and how we might want to celebrate this journey.
>
> In honour of breastfeeding, my daughter chose two special presents. First, she wanted a necklace made from my breastmilk. Together we studied several websites dedicated to breastmilk jewellery, and she picked out a design that appealed to her. Along with the breastmilk itself, she requested the inclusion of the birthstone that we share.

When she received the necklace, she was very excited, and she has since proudly worn it on special occasions. She likes knowing she will always have some of my milk with her.

Her second present was a photo album dedicated to breastfeeding. I included dozens of breastfeeding photos: her first feed, our first time feeding in public, us feeding in swimming pools and at the beach, feeding on a mountain and in a forest, feeding in cars and aeroplanes and on trains, feeding in countries around the world, tandem feeds with her younger sister, and some of her last feeds. Sometimes we look at this album together and reminisce about our experiences over the years, while other times she prefers to study it on her own; it seems to cheer her up during difficult moments.

Having these tangible reminders of our breastfeeding journey and our bond helped us cope with the bittersweet feeling we had about finishing breastfeeding. It will be interesting to see what celebratory gifts my younger daughter chooses when it's her turn to stop. (Woodstein 2022)

Woodstein has created a rite of passage for her family that gives space for contemplation and reflection. Note how her daughter is not being treated or rewarded for consenting to end breastfeeding. This is not, 'Well done for being such a good girl for not being sad anymore', or 'Let's have a party to celebrate ending breastfeeding'. I have seen discussions online of weaning parties with breast-shaped cakes and balloons: such events require great care. For a young child, a party is a happy event associated with joy and pleasure. Are we allowing the complex feelings that come with the end of breastfeeding? Do they understand that we are not expecting them to be happy? For some, this is time not so much for a party as a wake. It may be more suitable to have a shared experience where there is time and space to share memories and discuss feelings. Is that a celebration of weaning? We are not suggesting a parent provides a special day out as a 'treat' for accepting the ending of breastfeeding or a 'reward' for being a good boy and not complaining and protesting. Psychotherapist Amanda Joyce-Leon (@thedoulamanda) says we need to be wary of our 'toxic positivity culture' where a 'positive mindset' is always the ultimate goal. As they have all along the journey with their child, a parent will need to hold space for the sad and difficult feelings too. Some end-of-weaning celebrations are possibly motivated by guilt and are a form of guilt apology. Even at the end of the process, some parents haven't forgiven themselves for weaning and a 'special day' is another way to say sorry. It is possible to mark a goodbye to breastfeeding, without that being perceived as 'Let's be happy about weaning!'

Chapter 8

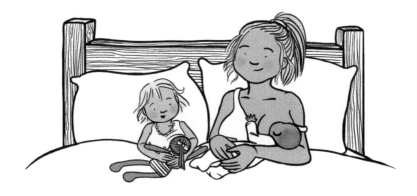

Weaning alongside a Partner

Families will often ask how the non-breastfeeding parent can help in the process. On rare occasions, weaning may be happening because of pressure from a partner. In extreme cases, we may be dealing with coercion or, certainly some firm persuading. The partner may even have strong ideas about a time frame or techniques that should be used, but their ideas are always secondary to the members of the breastfeeding dyad. Here are two people who are changing their relationship (the breastfeeding parent and the nursling). Only they can work through the transition together. They will both be learning new skills. A nursling needs to practise different forms of co-regulation and ways to ask for connection. A mother will be removing her prized parenting tool from her tool belt and putting it away forever. She has some upskilling to do that will come from trying new things and practising. A partner can provide valuable emotional support for both members of the partnership.

A supportive partner is key during the planning process. During the observation stage, when a feeding parent is reflecting on their child's motivation for feeding, a third party is a useful addition to the research team. They may well notice that requests come at a certain time before dinner when the feeding parent is on the phone, when a nap hasn't gone well earlier in the day or when the child feels socially overwhelmed. They may help a mother make connections and see things with fresh eyes. They can also help a feeding parent reflect on their options. It may not be that the issue is breastfeeding but the intensity of parenting a toddler, and additional support is needed. Has the feeding parent lost their ability to centre on themself? Is it time for some time away? Is it time for a mother to permit herself to put some boundaries in place? These conversations take time and, hopefully, a partner isn't going anywhere.

A partner can support a nursling too. Before weaning, it's valuable to have regular conversations about breastfeeding. An older child may also begin to notice their cues for wanting a feed. Hilary Flower quotes Bianca from Ohio: 'We try to talk about the difference between heart hungry and tummy hungry. While nursing can help heart hunger, there are other things we can do: snuggle, read a story, play dolls, etc.' (Flower 2019, p.155). It is helpful to talk about the fact that breastfeeding does end for everyone. Both parents can lead these conversations. This is not to say we are encouraging 'Big boys don't have mummy milk' chats, but conversations that explain that one day booby goes away, and it might be hard to say goodbye and they may need help. We can also encourage explicit conversations around other co-regulation and self-regulation methods. There might be a role play game where mummy teddy isn't giving booby milk anymore. How can we help baby teddy fall asleep? Both members of the dyad will be losing out on oxytocin and need some extra cuddles.

After a difficult night of putting new boundaries in place, it might be that the non-breastfeeding parent is on breakfast duty. They wake up fresh (or fresher) and have put some additional thought into offering an appealing breakfast and some activities that provide connection and affection. The breastfeeding parent may appreciate some additional time to sleep in.

What about the partner doing more than they usually do in terms of night time care? Is this the time to hand bedtime over to Daddy? Is this the time for the co-parent to take over night-time parenting entirely while the parent with the working breasts sleeps in another room with ear plugs, or even leaves the home entirely? Regularly, parents are presented with options like this when weaning comes into the conversation. Culturally, we accept abruptness and withdrawal as valid weaning methods. We sometimes hear of parents being told to simply leave their children to cry. These are families who have practised responsive breastfeeding and gentle parenting for years. Just as parents are often told that controlled crying and sleep training based around abandonment are the only ways to change sleep habits, they are often told that leaving a child is the only way to change their habits around breastfeeding. We hear of parents being told to walk away.

In her book *Milk: An Intimate History of Breastfeeding*, Joanna Wolfarth describes her choices around night weaning:

> So, we night weaned using a method women have used for centuries: abrupt absence. Children fed by their birth mothers would be removed to stay with grandparents, or the mother would stay elsewhere while the father stayed with the infant. And so, without warning, my mum and my husband sent me to a hotel for two nights. I put my son to bed, packed a small bag, and cried all the way to the bus stop. Halfway across London, the tears stopped, and my shoulders relaxed. By the time I was at the budget hotel I had acquired wine and snacks and, soon after, I luxuriated in solitude and sleep. At home, my baby woke up and cried. For a while. And then he slept through two nights, in bed beside my partner. The night-time spell was broken, and I started to gather the shards of my sanity. (2023, p.239)

Wolfarth clearly feels she made a decision that was right for her family (although this was not a full weaning experience) and it worked! It is likely they already had a family set-up where Daddy was a part of night-time care and there was a continuation of a familiar situation. Abrupt absence does not work for everyone, however, especially when someone who has previously not been responsible for night-time care takes over. In some cases, a parent returns and is leapt upon with a renewed enthusiasm for breastfeeding and a little person who is very determined to not fall for the same trick again. In some cases, because there has been no warning or preparation, there is a concern that Mummy may disappear again, and we can see a phase of a form of separation anxiety (which breastfeeding is great at solving). We can also find that when the parent does return and is back to night-time parenting, they are now beginning the process of introducing different forms of co-regulation layered on top of dealing with the emotional effects of their absence. Not every child will sleep through in response to this approach. For older children, we want to be as authentic as possible. The end of breastfeeding usually needs a warning.

I spoke to doula and psychotherapist Amanda Leon-Joyce about the need to face the difficult emotions of weaning head-on and why a 'drastic push away' may not be the answer:

> We had babies, but we are raising adults. As an adult, how would we want this person to experience a very significant ending? Would we want them to have a warning? Would we want someone to give them a hug and tell them they will be okay? Would we want them to be left alone? How would we want an adult to be supported through a significant ending? Because we can model that right now. The 'unworked-on' parts of ourselves can feel vulnerable in this process. We can subconsciously push that vulnerability onto our children and make them take the extra suffering that we are not able to take. We don't want to have a difficult conversation about an ending, so we push that difficult conversation away and increase what they need to carry, by making that ending then a surprise for them as well. It's such a touchy subject because nobody wants to make anyone feel worse about an ending. However, the difficulty can't be removed. It can just be moved... We might like to imagine that they are young and they forget but they won't. There is then a loss but no framework or understanding for that loss. At a preverbal stage, especially, there is no place to put that. Preverbally, everything is straight to the body. It doesn't mean the memories aren't there. They are just coded in body and not in words. We can't say for sure this is damaging but would we want to be treated that way? (Leon-Joyce 2022)

Weaning is 'the first grief, the first death, the first break-up'. Those strong feelings can't be walked away from. We cannot close the door to avoid facing them. As a family unit, how will difficult things be handled? Does this mean that a breastfeeding mother can never leave her child? Of course not. Wolfarth's break in a hotel sounds like a dream for someone struggling with sleep deprivation. A break like that might happen with an explanation and warning. It might be more sensible for a parent to have a break like that *prior* to starting a weaning process with an older child to catch up on sleep and have the necessary reserves, rather than as *part* of the weaning process. Many breastfeeding mothers go on work trips, visit unwell family members and work night shifts. They go on hen nights and stay with friends. Breastfed children are cared for lovingly by co-parents and other family members every day around the world.

Abrupt weaning often happens because a mother feels desperate. It also happens when we live in a world where parents struggle to get support as they breastfeed older children. They continue in isolation and then suddenly snap when it gets too much. If a mother is at breaking point, perhaps she needs time away to rest and relax and consider her options. How does she feel about breastfeeding on her return? If she is unable to leave, a period of greater support might help. She may then have the reserves to make a plan. Is there a way to consider how this feels from the child's perspective? When they are about to lose something precious to them, something that they have never lived without, who would they want to support them through that? If the breastfeeding parent walks away, who is that easier for? Weaning from breastfeeding should not feel like the loss of a parent. It is the loss of one thing a parent can do, and they are going to need to be there to make it very clear that there are lots of other things they *can* do. Abrupt absence is on par with putting an unpleasant tasting substance on nipples. It's an avoidance. Ideally, rather than avoiding difficult emotions, as psychotherapist Philippa Perry says, we want to be 'steering into the skid' of difficult feelings (Perry 2020, p.69).

If we are supporting a parent, and they declare that they wish to use an abrupt absence method, we cannot assume that they have not thought all their options through, but as breastfeeding supporters, we would support them to reflect on what happens after the separation. What problems have been solved? What problems might be created? What still needs to happen? All weaning methods can be considered as falling into three groups: 'likely to/may cause harm', 'unlikely to cause harm' and 'we don't know if it will cause harm'. We are creating a new relationship with the nursling, not simply removing a source of liquid. When a relationship is at the heart of this process, the child needs to feel safe, loved and validated. It's difficult to see how walking away helps that process unless a child is old enough to be a consenting collaborator with a full understanding of time periods and what is happening. When we challenge the technique of abrupt absence, we may provoke a parent's anger. There may even be parents who find my words here provoking. As breastfeeding supporters, we can absorb that anger, and help parents understand where it comes from and what it might represent. We are not therapists, but we can support parents to think through their methods and consider why they want to absent themselves from supporting their child to say goodbye to breastfeeding. It may be because they do not know what other methods are available. If their child fully understood what was happening, what would they ask for? There may be times when parents are at breaking point and *staying* might cause more harm, and we need to be sensitive to that. We are working with parents who are sleep deprived and desperate. Something that seems fast, and that their friends and family are pushing for and normalizing, is going to be very appealing. The possibility of walking away could mean a fix in a matter of days, but it may not be the fix that they were hoping for.

Sometimes the non-breastfeeding parent may be finding a child's emotional response difficult. This is a family that may never have seen a full emotional meltdown before. Offering the breast was always an option. At night, they may have never heard more than a murmur. The breastfeeding parent attached a nursling while hardly waking up. When it's 4 am and a child has been asking for the breast for 40 minutes (with lots of validation and love and cuddles), a partner may be tempted to think, 'Is this really worth it?' They may even feel like saying that. In complete opposition to the parents who put pressure on their partner to wean are those who put pressure on their partner to *not* wean. This is an issue of body autonomy. A mother has a right to decide when her breastfeeding experience will end and, ideally, their partner is there as their co-pilot, providing a loving safe space for all members of the family.

It is worth mentioning that sometimes a breastfeeding parent can fall into a pattern of 'always doing the bedtimes and night-time parenting'. After several years, they can be at breaking point and weaning feels like the only solution to that. Sometimes the partner's support can mean a continuation of breastfeeding in a new phase of parenting. There is no reason why, instead of losing breastfeeding entirely, a pre-schooler can understand that *this* is the night that Mummy gets extra sleep and 'you are with me' instead. We will miss Mummy, but Mummy needs to get some extra rest. Breastfeeding parents *can* go out at night. Nurslings *can* learn to fall asleep in different ways – sometimes. I'm also a big advocate of non-bedtime bedtime. Mummy can go out to yoga or to see friends and the nursling has a sofa picnic with the other caregiver. There is no need for the high pressure of trying to get them to bed if they are very breast dependent. Lights are dimmed, snuggles and books and hanging out happen, with the promise that 'Mummy will put you to bed when she gets back'. Usually, the nursling will fall asleep on the sofa anyway.

The true contribution a partner can make to the weaning conversation is to step back and help look at the bigger picture. That might mean asking some difficult questions about the patterns the family has fallen into. We need to check that the desire to end breastfeeding isn't coming from a desperate place that is really about the burden of caring for a young child and a home. What will change when breast-feeding ends? Are there things that a non-breastfeeding parent can do differently? How can a family best meet everyone's needs?

Chapter 9

Weaning in a Tandem Feeding Situation

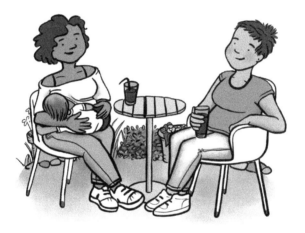

Most women who breastfeed will experience their periods returning at around 9–18 months (La Leche League International 2021). For some, it may be as soon as just a few weeks after birth, despite exclusive and frequent breastfeeding. There is a big range of normal. One study found that, among mothers breastfeeding responsively, the average return is 14.6 months (Kippley and Kippley 1972). The return to full fertility can vary greatly. Some will 'catch the first egg' and be pregnant without their menstrual cycle ever resuming. Others will have a regular monthly bleed but may have a short luteal phase (the gap between ovulation and the first day of the cycle). This means an implanted fertilized egg may not have sufficient time to build up the necessary hormone profile to inhibit the onset of the next period.

Whatever someone's circumstances, a lot of parents get pregnant again while breastfeeding. There are some aspects to the experience that will be universal. Everyone who has a pregnancy that reaches the second trimester will experience their milk resetting to colostrum (around 16 weeks). Even when the most enthusiastic toddler breastfeeder is part of the story, the pregnancy drives ahead with prioritizing newborn lactation and ensuring colostrum is available after birth. Colostrum does not taste the same as full-term regular milk, and quantities are very often smaller. If a nursling is drinking a considerable amount, their stools may become softer as the laxative effect of colostrum kicks in.

There are experiences which may not be universal. Some breastfeeding or chest-feeding parents experience nipple sensitivity and discomfort due to the hormonal changes of pregnancy. Some develop feelings of aversion and agitation that can bring considerable distress. Even when aversion doesn't develop, a parent may struggle with sleep during pregnancy and find that their tolerance for toddler breastfeeding behaviour has significantly reduced.

Some nurslings will happily continue to breastfeed throughout pregnancy, whatever is going on with the milk. If the parent experiences a reduction in volume, which most do, some nurslings will be outraged, and some will barely seem to notice. As Hilary Flower reminds us, 'Children are complex creatures, and their relationship to breastfeeding is many-layered' (Flower 2019, p.144). Some children may have been close to ending breastfeeding anyway and the pregnancy changes were a final trigger. Self-weaning during pregnancy may be abrupt if the motivation is a change in taste. Usually, self-weaning is described as a gradual process but when usually-sweet milk reduces in lactose content and becomes more savoury, 'children can sound like haughty restaurant critics as they give the thumbs down' (Flower 2019, p.144). Hilary Flower's book is an excellent resource for any parent and any professional supporting breastfeeding through pregnancy. It is comprehensive and supportive and will help parents to make informed decisions about their next steps.

If a child appears enthusiastic to continue, and the parent is not experiencing discomfort, breastfeeding may continue beyond pregnancy; and once the baby is born, the siblings might share – known as tandem nursing. It is called triandem feeding when twins are involved or there are two older nurslings. When a breastfeeding mum becomes pregnant, there is often a flood of emotions. One of those emotions can be guilt. They may be worried about the impact of the pregnancy on their breastfeeding relationship and worry that their child will be forced to end breastfeeding prematurely. They might be concerned that tandem feeding will bring increased stress to life with two children. Won't it increase jealousy? Won't the toddler/older child resent sharing their milk? Some parents may feel it's sensible to wean, but it is very difficult to make that decision based on a vision of a hypothetical life that you can have no realistic sense of. Some also feel an additional sense of panic because they fear that if weaning is too close to birth, they have committed the ultimate parenting sin. If a nursling is struggling with the weaning process, and then a baby comes along who breastfeeds all day long, the nursling's pain will surely be magnified significantly.

The decision of whether to wean during pregnancy is not something a parent has to rush. There is an extra charge to emotions when additional hormones come on the scene, and we need to try to engage with both sides of the brain before doing anything hasty. A key question is, how does breastfeeding feel right now: at this moment, this week, this month? If it is working for both of you and bringing positives, and the idea of saying goodbye to *this* breastfeeding feels tough, let's suggest a pause before assuming weaning is needed. Some parents encounter the historical myth that breastfeeding during pregnancy can be harmful to the pregnancy. I discussed this in more detail in my book *Supporting Breastfeeding Past the First Six Months and Beyond: A Guide for Professionals and Parents* (Pickett 2022, ch.9). The evidence is clear that breastfeeding 'should pose no added risk of pregnancy loss once a pregnancy is clinically detectable' (Regan 2018), and when a mother's nutrition is normal, there is no risk to the development of the baby. Throughout human history, where pregnancy testing wasn't an option, pregnancy and breastfeeding were compatible, normal, expected and uneventful. Evolution has meant that we can get pregnant while breastfeeding. Why would it make sense for something so catastrophic to happen to so many? It works.

Truthfully, tandem feeding after the baby arrives works for many too. Breastfeeding delivers a dose of oxytocin, the love and bonding hormone, just when a household needs it. Imagine speaking to a friend who is living with a newborn and a toddler and experiencing that post-birth chaos, and explaining to them that a legal drug exists that can transform everything. You are allowed to give your toddler this drug whenever you want throughout the day and night. You can also give it to your baby and even take it yourself (and your partner too). This drug has been proven to aid sleep and help everyone get back to sleep at night. It also affects your emotional state and has been shown to help new families bond and potentially help your older child to have loving feelings towards their new sibling. That drug would be the toast of the town. In a tandem breastfeeding situation, a parent has it. A breastfeed is a magic way to help a confused toddler regulate, keep calm and re-engage. It can still them, which is why the German word for breastfeeding – *stillen* – makes so much sense. They are naturally going to experience jealousy when a new sibling arrives. I once heard someone vividly describe the process of a new baby coming home as being like a husband telling his wife, 'Listen, I have a new wife. There's nothing you can do about it. She's coming to live with us. Forever. And you are going to love her.'

Does a parent really imagine that ending breastfeeding in advance is going to reduce jealousy? Based on what logic? Your arms, your gaze, your love and your time are still going to be an issue. And you may lose out on the value of that amazing drug (and there's more than one) just when you need it. I need to declare a personal bias here. I can do this confidently in the knowledge my children will be very unlikely to read this far. My now 18-year-old son has a beautiful relationship with his 15-year-old sister: loving, kind and supportive. I believe deep in my maternal soul (and my IBCLC (International Board Certified Lactation Consultant) soul) that their experience of tandem feeding after my daughter's birth set them off on a path that forged that positive relationship. I also believe that nature isn't daft. What a clever system when a new family is creating a new life for itself! That's not to say that I won't regularly be supporting parents to end breastfeeding in pregnancy, but it takes some reflection to ensure a decision is being made for the right reasons and not from a place of panic. Sometimes, the panic exists because they feel night-time parenting has to change. They believe they have to end breastfeeding so that co-sleeping can end, so a child can move into their room, and so the next baby's life can look like what we culturally expect a baby's life to look like.

This new baby's life will not be the same. The parents are not the same. The household is not the same. There is no reason why a family has to end co-sleeping if they don't feel ready for 'hypothetical baby world' reasons. Throughout most of human history moving older children into separate bedrooms wasn't even an option. Will their sleep be disturbed? It is surprising how often it won't be when a family is responsively breastfeeding and co-sleeping with a newborn. There are some safety guidelines (such as ensuring that a young child and newborn aren't sleeping next to each other), but there are all sorts of options that keep a family together and ensure safe sleeping guidance is followed.

That was a lot of information about not weaning, but it's important, as with any other weaning decision, that a choice to end breastfeeding is a choice coming from a place of informed motivation. Often when a parent wants to end breastfeeding during pregnancy, they were already on that road even before they were pregnant.

The process of ending breastfeeding during pregnancy may be eased by the reduction in supply and the taste change. In some cases, it can be used as an additional nudge. We want the conversation between parent and child to be as authentic as possible, but it can certainly help to have a practical demonstration of the milk 'going away'. If a parent says, 'My body is making less milk now and I'm going to need to help you have cuddles without milk', that can be a useful starting point. As we discussed in Chapter 7, every child has a different relationship to the breast and the parent is not simply taking away breastfeeding but ensuring that they are filling the hole with connections that meet their child's emotional needs, or their sleep or nutritional needs.

Some parents get the message that there is a window for weaning during pregnancy. They are told it shouldn't be too close to the birth or the risk is that the end of breastfeeding becomes associated with the baby, and the ex-nursling perceives their new sibling to have 'taken it'. When we investigate where this fear comes from, and the basis for it, it seems to be no more than 'it seems sensible'. But when have breast-feeding professionals based their practice on 'it seems sensible'? It is a simplistic view of the situation when there are a thousand factors to consider. Imagine the state of the mother who is considering weaning just a few weeks before she is due to give birth. She is likely speaking from a place of desperation, and to be met with, 'It's probably not a good idea now because of a theory that seems sensible' feels dismissive. What are we saying? That it is also not sensible to wean *after* the birth, so she could be looking at continuing for several months?

If a mother is struggling, she has the right to end breastfeeding whenever she chooses, and we can support her to do that. She can be as authentic as possible, but with no need to specifically talk about the baby needing milk and having to stop for that reason. Having said that, I'm not sure it is quite the evil we imagine to say, 'The new baby will need the milk now'. Do we believe that alone is going to cause resentment and difficulty? For some older children, that may be an enormous sense of pride and something that makes perfect logical sense. The very popular picture book *Booby Moon* is centred around that concept, and it can work. Siblings are often hardwired to want to care for 'their' babies.

Similarly, weaning soon after the baby arrives can also seem logical to an older nursling. Some parents are surprised that when they give birth, the older nursling suddenly seems out of place at the breast, and they may even experience aversion when feeding them for the first time. This might not resolve with time, and it may feel like weaning is the desired option. Another 'because it seems sensible' theory is that we are not supposed to change more than one thing at a time in the life of a young child. However, there can be times when combining more than one change feels natural. When supporting toddlers and pre-schoolers to wean, it is notable how many decide to end breast-feeding themselves when something else occurs – they stop wearing nappies during the day or they have moved into a big bed. They make an association themselves that feels logical. They may have been feeding out of habit, and when a habit shifts, it naturally falls always with no distress.

When a new baby has arrived, a lot of habits change. They may see breastfeeding in a different light. It can be useful for parents to highlight that the baby is dependent on breastfeeding, but the older child can have their needs met in lots of different ways. This can be physically demonstrated by creating a family pictogram. For young children, the concept of time is mostly abstract, but we can try to represent their breastfeeding experience in a concrete way. A parent can take a large piece of paper and use a felt-tip pen to mark every month the older child has been breastfeeding (or every week or even every day if they have the time). They can then make felt-tip marks that represent their new baby sibling's experiences. If this has worked to plan, they should be immediately struck by just how many breast-feeding opportunities they have had in their life. They have had a fair shot. You could then, particularly for an older child, indicate all the weeks that they *only* had milk, and compare that to their baby sibling. It makes complete logical sense for even a toddler to understand that they can have other foods and the baby can't. For a younger child who may be going through a phase of exploring concepts of fairness and sharing, it makes sense to highlight that they have had a fair turn. It is possible to explain that it is time for breastfeeding to come to an end, even when a baby will still be continuing to breastfeed in the house.

As in any other situation, weaning is not simply the removal of breastfeeding but the need to consider what will fill the space. When there is a new baby in the house, it's a particularly helpful time to reflect on how the older child can connect with their mother/feeding parent. Even when a family isn't weaning, a conscious process of think-ing that through is sensible. The child may also be able to have some input. What would they like to do when they want to feel calm, cosy or the focus of attention? We want them to have some options that they have agency over and they can request. For a young child, that means labelling different options in a language they can use themselves.

Once the weaning process begins, there are different approaches. Hopefully, during pregnancy, some boundaries have already been put in place. I would not recommend anyone gives birth to a new baby when there is a toddler still breastfeeding in the house under 'Don't refuse / they are the boss' conditions. We want them to have already understood that sometimes Mummy feels tired, or sore. We want them to have experience role-playing life with the baby and to know that sometimes they may need to wait or help out. They might have a new place for sleeping. When the baby arrives, they may already be prepared for the idea that mummy milk only happens in the bedroom, or that it only happens a specific number of times a day, or only for 'count to ten'. During pregnancy, a parent will not be able to predict how life with two is going to feel. Tandem feeding (in the sense of actually feeding two simultaneously) may end up feeling very special. It might be the one time that they feel they can create some peace, or they may feel 'touched out' and want to speed up the process.

Most weaning picture books do not cater for a tandem feeding situation, but there is an exception: *Booby Moon with Two* by Yvette Reid, illustrated by Camilio Zepeda (Reid 2022). The book explains that once the baby is here, there will be a period of tandem nursing: 'For a while we will share, we each will have a side' (2022, p.9). However, that period will end, 'And as I grow, I'll nurse much less. My heart will fill with pride' (p.10). The older sibling letting the baby nurse is presented as being 'kind' and showing how much he cares. They then let the booby moon float away using the symbol of a balloon, as happens in Yvette Reid's *Booby Moon: A Weaning Book for Toddlers* (2021). However, there is space after that for more difficult feelings. The older sibling feels sad and even has pangs when the baby is feeding. Mama needs to find other ways for them to connect. It's helpful to have recognition of the fact that sadness is going to be a normal part of this process, and this is not about expecting happy compliance. Even feelings of jealousy might be normal and should be supported, rather than imagining they can be avoided. On first reading, this book might make you nervous that the sibling is expected to give up the breast merrily as part of being 'kind' to the baby, but there is space for a full range of emotions. The book ends with a quote from A.A. Milne (1926, quoted in Reid 2022), which sums up this whole weaning experience: 'How lucky am I to have something that makes saying goodbye so hard'. The book also contains a user guide which gives helpful suggestions and has a link to connect with other parents on Facebook.

If we don't support parents to end breastfeeding at whatever time feels needed, what is the alternative? Continuing while feeling distressed and resentful at the very time they need all their emotional reserves? The changes in milk provide a natural transition in pregnancy and many nurslings will only require an extra nudge. The concept that weaning is out of bounds when there is a new baby in the house misses the point that some nurslings themselves start to see breastfeeding in a new light and even declare that milk is for the baby now. Far from it being an impossibility, the arrival of a new baby can be a logical hook that provides a clear and simple explanation for the end of breastfeeding. When routines are shaken up, a new daily routine that focuses on other ways of connecting can be easier to introduce.

Chapter 10

Weaning Led by the Child

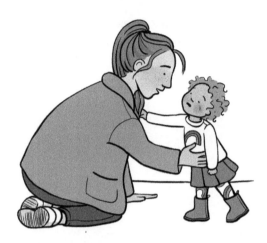

Professionals who are regularly supporting families breastfeeding past infancy, and spending time within the community online, will be familiar with the phrase 'self-weaning'. It is sometimes called 'natural-term weaning', but that would be an incorrect phrasing. If we take the natural term of breastfeeding for humans to be around three to seven years, then any weaning that takes place in that time frame, whether child-led or parent-nudged, would surely fit the definition. Self-weaning or child-led weaning refers to breastfeeding that ends when a child is ready. The nursling is in control and the parent respects their wishes.

Unsurprisingly, the concept of self-weaning is not well studied but most breastfeeding professionals seem to agree on a few parameters. The child 'is typically well over a year old (more commonly, over two years), is at the point where he gets most of his nutrition from solids, drinks well from a cup, [and] cuts down on nursing gradually' (Bonyata 2022).

If breastfeeding ends abruptly and hasn't been gradually tapered down, then a family may be dealing with other factors such as a nursing strike, a temporary response to illness or other factors affecting the relationship to the breast such as a reduction in milk supply. When I asked parents for their stories of self-weaning, it was notable how many accounts did not fit the accepted definition. Some parents had already practised parent-led night weaning or had been putting other boundaries in place. However, they perceived the end of the breast-feeding relationship as self-weaning for their child. In some cases, nurslings were significantly below 12 months and had developed a preference for the bottle. In a world where parent-led weaning isn't often discussed, and self-weaning is seen as the goal, it's not unex-pected when parents would prefer to feel their own experience can be awarded this label.

In reality, 'pure' child-led weaning is not an attainable experience in the vast majority of cases, and holding it up as the goal may be unhelpful. There is always a spectrum. Along the way, parents intro-duce solid food. They offer cups with other fluids and sometimes other kinds of milk. They go out for the evening or even away for a weekend. They return to work and their child is cared for by other adults who settle them to sleep in different ways. They sometimes postpone a feed because they have to eat something or go to the toilet. As nurslings grow older, negotiation becomes normal. Sometimes parents feel like cuddling instead or would prefer not to feed in a particular location at a particular time. Any negotiation is a parental nudge in the direc-tion of weaning. Weaning for many families is a series of interactions spread over an extended time where slowly and gently the dependence on the breast changes. It is difficult to write the definition of child-led weaning in stone. Deciding what is 'true' self-weaning is only useful when we are supporting a family through a nursing strike. How does the parent feel about their child rejecting the breast and not wanting to feed? What was the breastfeeding pattern before this? From what they are describing, it doesn't sound as though their child was tapering off feeding gradually, and this is probably a temporary phase. How can we support them next?

Another area for support is helping parents to understand what is normal. A parent who is struggling with breastfeeding an 18-month-old, and desperately hoping that their nursling (who breastfeeds throughout the night and regularly during the day) is going to self-wean soon, can benefit from hearing other experiences of the gradual tapering-off of breastfeeds as a child takes the lead. It can be helpful to say that although self-weaning doesn't look the same for everyone, there are some common threads, and if a parent is hoping for self-weaning soon, that's a clue that they may need support to put some boundaries in place. If a parent finds themself scouring the internet looking for stories that confirm their dream that early self-weaning *does* happen, they may be struggling to care for themselves in the face of believing that self-weaning is the goal all good parents aspire to.

Liz's story reminds us to be cautious around strict age parameters. Is this a mother nudging a child along and retrospectively defining it as self-weaning? I don't believe it is.

My second breastfed like a dream. It was like she'd read the book. No weight loss, a real chunky thing, perfect latch. As she was my last baby, I was planning to feed her until she stopped. I'd not set any time limit to that. By 12 months old she'd naturally dropped all but two feeds. By the start of the pandemic and 14 months old she was only having a morning feed. One day at 17 months she flatly refused that morning feed. She wanted a cup of milk just like her big brother. The next morning the same. Every morning when I offered, she refused. She had decided enough was enough. As much as I wanted to be led by her, I was sad as in my own mind I'd expected to get to two years at least. I felt like I was failing her in some way because I hadn't done the full time I'd intended to.
(Liz)

Alida describes a typical end to breastfeeding with some give and take on both sides:

I always wanted to let my daughter take the lead with weaning, as my mum did with me. She was a total 'boob monster' and, for want of a better phrase, a 'terrible sleeper' so it seemed to me to be the easier option rather than imposing routines and generally fighting against what she wanted/needed. We co-slept from when she was around four months old (C-section healing meant I didn't do it from birth), which meant she had unlimited open booby bar access through the night. I thought we'd be feeding forever, which I wouldn't have minded massively. When my daughter turned three, her sleep suddenly improved. I think this was because her teeth were all through. She fed far less in the night, and less in the day. Bearing in mind this was during Covid lockdowns, I was working from home, so again, generally, she had open access to the booby bar. Her feeding frequency gradually decreased until she was only really interested at bedtime, which again got less and less frequent and for a shorter time each time. By this time, she was in full-time nursery school, so busy all day and only occasionally wanting to feed when she came home. Eventually, she started going to sleep without 'boobs' as she called it. By this time my supply was decreasing and eventually dried up, so there was nothing for her to have.

Prior to the decreasing, I started to find I had an aversion, mostly around the time of my period being due. So, I'd occasionally limit the time she was latched on if it got a bit toe curling. Sometimes she'd feed more frequently if she had a cold or something, but generally, it decreased. Once she did stop (that is, it had been weeks and weeks), I felt pretty OK with this. We'd had an amazing run getting to three-and-a-half years, I was ready to stop, as was she. I did and do still occasionally miss breastfeeding as a tool for comfort, particularly if she's hurt herself. But she's still super-cuddly and attached, and still obsessed with mentioning or touching my boobs at any opportunity. Again, I'm working on boundary setting here as it gets a bit much for me at times, being 'touched out'. I'm extremely proud of our journey and wouldn't change it for the world. She still sleeps in my bed; we're still just as close.

(*Alida*)

Poppy's account is a reminder that comments from other relatives may sometimes have a role in a child deciding to stop breastfeeding. The feeding parent may not always be aware it is even happening:

Feeding had been gradually reducing over the last 18 months, to predominantly bedtime feed, or if she was unwell/upset. I had a medical procedure a few months before and we had a few days of no nursing and I thought that was it, but then she asked again at bedtime. So we were back to bedtime, often just for a few minutes. In the last two months, it was getting less consistent, and I would sometimes ask if she wanted to feed. She started saying she didn't so we started talking about it and she was saying she was a big girl and was starting school later in the year and so she didn't need it (I think my mother-in-law put those thoughts/words in her head though), so we talked about her deciding when it was the last feed, which she just announced one evening. We had a picture of her nursing and then a lovely hug, and that was it. She still (now eight years old) remembers she was breastfed and talks lovingly of it. It was a lovely natural end that felt right (albeit a bit sad and unnerving to think how to parent without it!).

(*Poppy*)

Sometimes a partner is the one providing the nudge; Carolyn:

My kids were breastfed until they were four and five. With three years between them, that included a year breastfeeding both. I felt quite strongly that they should breastfeed until they no longer wanted to. I must say we did begin to wonder if that moment would ever come naturally, to our son in particular, and used to joke of the somewhat unsettling vision of a bearded grown man with a deep voice asking me for 'bap'! I never got the urge that some friends did to have them finish with the breast, and so as long as they wanted to, I was happy to; in fact, I treasured these moments of quiet connection. I felt they got much more from breastfeeding than mere milk. They were comforted and soothed at the breast. The last year or two would be just at bedtime or at times of great upset, like when they hurt themselves. I would say my partner was not comfortable with it in the same way that I was, and his mum and sister were certainly not.

Near to his fourth birthday, Saul (who had been sleeping on a little extension we built onto the side of our bed) announced that he would like a bunk bed. His dad immediately said that he would be big enough to have one when he was four and that he would build him one, but big boys who sleep in bunk beds don't have 'bap'. And that was that. On the eve of his fourth birthday, he consciously drank his last. It felt quite momentous! The next few nights were really hard for him as this had been his way to fall asleep, but we decided that he could hold the breast instead, which he did, and I sang, and he did drop off in the end. I felt sad in some ways and proud of him also, and he was thrilled with his bunk bed. His younger sister Anaya stopped at nearly five. It's funny but my memory of how it ended is fuzzy. I think this is because she wasn't coerced in any way, and it dropped naturally. She made the decision and I remember using the 'holding technique' with her also. I'm so grateful to have had this precious time with them.
(*Carolyn*)

Rebecca's experience shows how both mother and child may go through phases and the relationship with breastfeeding can change:

I would have happily stopped at any point after two years but as Covid hit, and understanding the amazingness that is breastmilk, and antibodies, combined with the lack of a social life, we carried on. My son has only fed at bedtime for quite some time – probably since about 18 months. At age two he decided he didn't want to bother with one boob, so I continued to feed off one side. When he turned three, I started to consider weaning more. But then I realized that there were really no cons to continuing to breastfeed. Up to that age he had breastfed to sleep every night within ten minutes. If I wasn't there he would happily lie in bed while my husband or mum sat with him. I was not tied to bedtime, but boy did breastfeeding make it easy!

Just before he turned four, he started skipping mummy milks and opting to go straight to bed. Despite being fed to sleep the majority of his first four years, he now settles in bed and goes to sleep with a few check-ins for cuddles. We spoke about stopping feeding when he was four but this was me planting the seed rather than forcing it. I employed, 'Don't offer, Don't refuse', but I was also aware after a number of days to let him know the mummy milk might stop working. This always prompted him to feed and we were probably feeding once or twice a week. After a couple of months of this, I decided to see if he would draw a line under it if we spoke about it. With his agreement, we said bye to the mummy milks. He wasn't at all upset. He did ask twice after this (and so I agreed as I wanted to be led by him ultimately), but he only fed for a couple of seconds. It was well over a month of no feeds before I felt I could say we had stopped. It has certainly been really odd. Natural-term weaning has meant a lot of uncertainty in some ways, but it has also been so lovely to follow his lead. I can't remember our final feed, but I have many photos from along the way. Not many people know that I breastfed for so long. I am not embarrassed by it, but I am equally aware how hard it can be to understand unless you have experienced it.

(Rebecca)

Kirsty's experience reminds us that ending breastfeeding doesn't necessarily result in a child sleeping through the night:

We had been doing a mixture of direct breastfeeding and expressed breast milk for a while as grandparents had been helping with childcare. Daytime feeds had stopped, probably about a month before as she was eating enough solid food to maintain her and enjoyed drinking water and cow's milk if offered. Night-time feeds continued for comfort more than anything. Then we went through a funny stage where she would wake in the night to play: she didn't want milk; she was wide awake and happy for a few hours in the middle of the night. At this stage, we ended up sleeping on her floor while she played, and she would eventually fall asleep on her own. That was a really tough period in terms of lack of sleep, but ultimately it ended in her sleeping through the night and weaning herself. The sleeping through the night didn't last long; she's four now and still occasionally wakes, but other forms of comfort were enough to settle her again. I feel sad that I don't remember the last feed we had though; it wasn't a conscious decision, it just happened organically. *(Kirsty)*

Bethan's story represents the nudge that pregnancy can often bring. Around two-thirds of parents notice a drop in milk supply and everyone will reset to colostrum in the second trimester in preparation for the newborn. It is also common for nipple sensitivity and sometimes aversion to be an issue in pregnancy:

I am now 22 weeks pregnant, and my milk has all but disappeared. My boy, Max, had a little encouragement rather than it being truly child-led, but due to his age and understanding that the milk isn't really there anymore (including some daily 'checks' where he'd latch to see!) made the weaning process very easy. I [validated his feelings when he expressed] that it is sad, and I said I've enjoyed feeding him too. I flagged that breastfeeding ends for everyone, and asked the family how they get to sleep without boobie. We also discussed how he might like to get to sleep without feeding. After about four weeks of this, he dropped daytime feeds and the morning feed without any pushing and only a tiny bit of me suggesting we'd wait until later instead. Another week or two after, he was having a little check feed to see if there was milk before bed and coming off the breast himself to fall asleep. He took a little further encouragement to drop the little dry nursing before sleep and now goes to sleep without asking for milk and without being upset. Bedtimes are taking a little longer as feeding to sleep was like a magic button, but it's still a big adaption and early days. He's doing so well and I'm glad we kept going with the flow until now. I don't feel sad about the journey ending as we had a good run and the end seems natural, relaxed and understood by Max.

(**Bethan**)

Sophie's story represents how the ending isn't always clear. Many parents don't know when the last feed was and 'the last feed' can extend over a surprisingly long time:

My daughter is four and a few months. I always intended to let her come to a natural end of breastfeeding. Over the last few months (maybe even longer, like six months) is when I noticed more of a natural progression towards much less feeding than before. So, it was just a really gradual thing. Where once boobie was still there to soothe big emotions or connect or whatever the reason, it became less, with no involvement on my part. Gradually she would breast-feed to sleep only but started going some nights where she would just cuddle. At times she would have it still if she was poorly. But more recently there has been a definite lack of asking at all, and even declining if offered – 'no thanks'. She became happy just having my arm to lay on at bedtime. The strange thing is she very very infrequently still asks for it. She has a couple of sucks and then says there's no milk. This has been happening for maybe a month now, so I feel like she has weaned but still has these random episodes. I bought a book to read to her on weaning to celebrate our journey.

I know for me over the last few months I have had waves of grief at the end of this incredible journey. But when we read the book, she said she still isn't saying goodbye to mummy's milk, as though she is still a bit in between. But when I point out, 'You never have it!', she says she does, so I guess she is maybe still processing this change. And maybe I'm hanging on a bit too. I'm so proud to have nursed her for four years and I think I will still be reliving memories of this for a while and still coming to terms with it, as she may be. Ending it so gradually and on her terms has been a really lovely process to go through.
(*Sophie*)

Sarah's story shows how the line between a nursing strike and self-weaning can be a blurry one:

My toddler had decreased his breastfeeds down to just the evening and in the night if he woke up, although some wake-ups had just become a cuddle. He contracted hand, foot and mouth, which caused a couple of blisters on his tongue, meaning he couldn't latch. I offered him the breast for three evenings and he would try, but come straight off and cuddle instead. Before this, he would ask for milk as soon as we started putting his jammies on but, since those three days, he never asked again. I found this tough because it wasn't planned, and I felt frustrated because it happened when he was poorly and I thought breast milk could help him recover quicker.
(*Sarah*)

It may have been possible to encourage feeding to resume, but Sarah's son was clearly heading for the door of his breastfeeding journey anyway. His experience with illness meant that the end was more abrupt than we might expect.

Brianna's son also ended breastfeeding quite abruptly, but in a way that made sense to him:

When he was three, we were talking about teeth. I am very matter of fact and I told him all his teeth would fall out and he would get his new ones, and they were already there. We got into a really big discussion about why he had those teeth and what his new teeth would be like, and why they are called milk teeth, and why his toothpaste is described as being 'for milk teeth'. We were talking about that a lot, and he said, 'So when I lose my first tooth, that's when I'll stop having "boop"'. That's what he decided. When he lost his first tooth, he was very upset, and he cried for quite a while. 'I've lost my tooth and now I can't have boop anymore!' I said we can talk about it, and he said, 'No, I can't. I said this and I must do this.' He was six. I was feeding the baby, and feeding him as well wasn't a bother, but he was adamant: 'I said it, so I must do it. That's what the science says!'
(Brianna)

Helena was also a bit taken aback by the end of her breastfeeding experience:

Having returned to work at ten months, I continued to breastfeed, but my daughter chose to remain exclusively breastfed despite my efforts to pump and also offer alternatives. This meant she would just wait for me to come home and feed overnight. From 15 months and onwards, she had started sleeping through the night more reliably and not needing a feed overnight, and was only having a feed before bedtime to help her get to sleep. One week before she turned 18 months, I had her ready for bed and she seemed to be reaching towards the cot. I gave her the choice to go in the cot or over to the chair where I would normally feed her, and she again reached for the cot. So I put her down and she went to sleep just like that. I left the room in a state of shock both elated that I could respect her choices and give her the time and space to make this decision on her own (despite significant challenges with her sleep), but also a little confronted that she hadn't chosen to have a feed. From then on, I chose not to reoffer at bedtime, and she didn't ask for it again. Had I known the previous night it would have been our last feed I think I would have felt all sorts of emotions, but, subsequently, on reflection, I can say with confidence I completely respected my daughter's feeding needs and her wishes from beginning to end (not without huge hurdles) for which I feel immensely proud of myself. *(Helena)*

Leigh-Ann and Kathy both describe a peaceful winding-down that is very much child-led.

Leigh-Ann:

I planned to breastfeed to natural term while I was pregnant with my daughter, and despite a very challenging start to our breast-feeding journey (which almost didn't get off the ground at all), I found that I was parenting through breastfeeding. It was my tool for everything: helping her to sleep, comforting when she was sad or poorly, or providing extra fluids during hot weather, as well as the perfect way to reconnect after a day apart when I'd been working. She stopped waking at night just before her third birthday. Before this time if I was there, she'd feed back to sleep, which was by far the quickest way to support her. If she was with her nanny, she'd have water and a back rub to help her back to sleep. For the next year, after she stopped waking overnight, her feeds gradually reduced. Sometimes when she was upset, I'd offer but she'd refuse. I noticed a gradual change in her relationship with her breastfeeding journey, as it became less important to her. For a few months, before she stopped completely, she would latch for around 10–30 seconds on one side (where previously it would have been both) and then unlatch before she was asleep, roll over and ask for a back rub to help her off to sleep. Shortly after her fourth birthday she latched on but seemed to struggle to get the right motion and angle and that was it. I offered the next night, but she wasn't interested and

just wanted a back rub to sleep. I'm so incredibly proud of allowing her to choose, and it felt very natural and easy for us, which I'll be eternally grateful for, but I'm not sure I was completely ready for it to end.
(*Leigh-Ann*)

Kathy:

The end of our breastfeeding journey was very gentle. He was down to one evening feed for about four months before it finished altogether. During the last month or so, I could sense my supply had dropped. The feeding suddenly started to feel different. In the lead-up to his self-weaning we had been through the toilet learning process. This was a big shift in how he saw himself, plus he started at a new nursery. One night he was so engrossed in bedtime stories with his dad that he didn't ask. This then repeated for the next few nights and marked the end of our beautiful journey together. I felt very emotional and reflective as it's probably the only breastfeeding experience I'll ever have. Wonderful memories I'll have forever.
(*Kathy*)

Charlotte's story reminds us of the potential impact when a parent receives messages that younger toddlers 'don't self-wean'. In fact, her daughter's story, with its gradual tapering off, would fit most people's definition of self-weaning, but the age didn't fit with what Charlotte had been taught in her training, and she was left with feelings of grief and confusion:

My daughter 'self-weaned' when she was 15 months old. I didn't see it coming; didn't imagine this chapter of mothering would end as it did. I can't remember our last feed. I do remember feeling initial relief. The freedom! And then crushing sadness as my hormones shifted, as I relearnt how to offer comfort and closeness, and as I started to process everything that our experience had been.

In the newborn days, breastfeeding was a great struggle. An early-term baby as I later learnt, born at 37 weeks, an undiagnosed tongue tie and a 'lazy' (at best) suck reflex meant triple-feeding, exclusive pumping and nipple shields. Navigating this during a global pandemic without the support I so desperately needed was hard, but I persevered, and we found our way together. Margot feeding from my breast seemed like the greatest blessing after the rocky start and I accepted the nipple shields were here to stay. No matter how many times I followed advice to 'pop them off mid-way through a feed', her little chubby hand would always madly thrash around looking for the familiar silicone she was so used to.

And then, when Margot was around 14 months old, she started to show less interest in feeding. Her appetite for solid foods had increased, and I put it down to simply needing less milk. But then the morning feed seemed to get shorter and shorter until she began to simply start the day without the fuss of a feed first. The bedtime feeds lasted the longest and then, slowly but surely, she found less comfort in the familiarity of feeding and would happily finish before falling asleep – instead wanting to be rocked and sang to. And before I knew it, that was the end.

And at the time, I assumed it was just her way. We joke about how stubborn she can be, and how well she knows her own mind. She's admirably determined and fiercely independent when she wants to be. I guessed she had decided she was done; and in the immediate days and weeks following that final feed I allowed myself to ignore the quiet whisperings of my intuition telling me there was more to it than that.

It was only when I trained as a Breastfeeding Peer Supporter that I started to tune into my instinct: factsheets telling me it's very unusual for a baby to self-wean before two years of age; the WHO recommending continued breastfeeding for up to two years and beyond. Something didn't feel quite right about how early our personal breastfeeding journey had ended. And so began the feelings of grief and of loss. Despite the trauma of breastfeeding in the early months, it's the lost second half of our experience that I grieve: the toddler years; the parenting tool I wish I'd had for so much longer; the benefits I could've given her, and me; the club I could've belonged to.

I feel lucky that I have been able to give myself the space I need to feel all of these feelings, plus the anger and frustration that I wasn't surrounded by knowledge and support that may have changed the outcome, and the regret that I didn't reach out to find a professional at the time. I will never know the reason that breastfeeding ended for us when it did. Could it have been frustration due to the nipple shields? Perhaps it was teething pain that I didn't pick up on. Or distraction as Margot's world grew? And for many, their child self-weaning is a relief – it gives them permission to stop, and I absolutely felt that too. Nothing needs to be binary, and these feelings will always have existed alongside the grief. It wasn't a sudden ending: nothing that would suggest a nursing strike or discomfort. It just felt like she started to find less and less comfort in the feeds – she didn't seem to fall asleep so easily, she didn't ever ask for a feed. I guessed she had just decided she was done. I'm angry there wasn't more information open to me through the whole of my breastfeeding journey. The ending clouds the rest sometimes. Babywearing helped. Margot still uses skin-to-skin for comfort. My chest and tummy are still her safe place.
(Charlotte)

You can hear how conflicted Charlotte still feels. Throughout the breastfeeding support world, every family's story is different, and as professionals, we must resist the temptation to put families into boxes and instead support everyone on an individual basis. Parents who experience self-weaning also need our support – to understand what's normal and to come to terms with the end of their breastfeeding experience. If anyone can understand what they might be feeling, and the complexities of those feelings, it will be us.

Chapter 11

Weaning When There Are Additional Needs

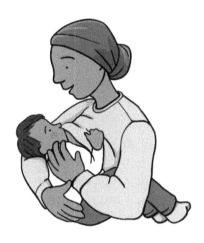

As described previously, parents often struggle to centre on themselves in the weaning conversation. 'Good' mothers don't put themselves first according to many cultural messages we receive throughout our lives. They continue with situations that may be uncomfortable or even painful if it meets their child's needs because 'that's what good parents do'. Some parents will choose to continue breastfeeding, even if they are not enjoying it and they wish it would end tomorrow, if they feel it is the best thing for their child. Sometimes the prospect of ending breastfeeding seems too challenging, and continuing reluctantly feels like the easier option. If a child has additional needs or medically complex needs, a parent is even less likely to put their feelings ahead of their child's. These parents need still greater support to find space for self-care and to permit themselves to consider the end of breast-feeding. These may be children who will benefit from a gradual and considered weaning process, so it is particularly valuable that a parent is supported along the process, rather than get themselves to a place of desperation where breastfeeding may end abruptly.

If a child has dietary needs that mean they are dependent on breastmilk, a parent may feel they have little choice but to continue breastfeeding. However, an older child may not be able to breastfeed indefinitely. As children get older, it can be harder to achieve an effective latch that means breastmilk is transferred optimally. The age at which this occurs seems to vary, but it seems to coincide for many with the loss of baby teeth and a change to the shape of the face and palate. Sometimes a child may report that they are struggling to get milk out despite all their best efforts. This phenomenon is not well studied, and there does not appear to be a universal experience, but it is sensible for any family who are continuing to breastfeed for nutritional reasons to be prepared in advance for changes to their circumstances and to have the right support in place if breastfeeding was to end.

Parents breastfeeding a child with additional needs require more support with weaning, even if the end may feel some way off because the process of ending breastfeeding requires more consideration and planning. In a family where the breastfeeding parent is autistic, they are often well informed about breastfeeding, having done a lot of personal research (Grant and Williams 2022). In turn, the breastfeeding supporter working with a family must be knowledgeable about how being autistic can affect a parent's feeding experience. There is inadequate feeding support for many families around the world. This is even more the case with autistic parents. It has sometimes been said in the past that autistic people lack empathy. As Dr Aimee Grant describes:

> This has been disproven, with part of the issue being, in fact, that often neurotypical people do not feel empathy towards Autistic people. This is known as the 'double empathy problem'. Even if you cannot begin to imagine what the Autistic person is telling you – for example

one person said that breastfeeding felt like having an old-fashioned telephone ringing in their breasts – please empathize with them. If they tell you something feels unbearable, but that they still want to continue breastfeeding, empathize with them first and then ask if they'd like to try to problem solve with you, rather than saying that formula is the only solution. Ask them what the worst thing is. It may be difficult for them to answer, so be patient and give them time to think. (Grant 2022)

It should be noted that autistic people may not all be happy with a phrase like 'additional needs' and may not wish to be described as 'having autism'. We should ask the parents we support about the language they prefer to use. Autistic people are not a homogeneous group. For many, autism is a positive thing:

> I don't see being autistic as 'having' a disorder. Instead, I look at it as a very positive thing. From a young age, it has helped me direct a laser-like focus on achieving my goals... 'Being autistic' rather than 'having autism' promotes the idea of difference, rather than disability.
> *(Ransom 2023)*

Everyone's lived experience will be different. In some homes, a young autistic child may be non-verbal, and their parents are going to need to work hard to provide other forms of regulation once breastfeeding ends. Conceiving the end of breastfeeding can be frightening. In other homes, autism may mean a parent is driven to make breastfeeding and weaning work and is highly focused and well informed, but does not wish to receive any breastfeeding advice over the phone and prefers to communicate via email.

I spoke to Becks Harper, who is an autistic parent and autistic parent supporter with a background in breastfeeding peer support:

Q: If a breastfeeding professional is working to support an autistic parent to end breastfeeding, what are some things you would like them to know about autism?

A: Being autistic is a variation from the assumed typical way a person's brain processes the world. The person you are supporting will likely experience the world around them differently from you. This is generally most noticeable to those around them in their sensory experiences and their social communication skills. The environment you are in will matter greatly in the success of your interaction. Ensure the parent is really comfortable with the space they are in: light, noise, furniture, where you're sitting in relation to each other. Check in with the parent!

An autistic person who is experiencing high levels of stress or anxiety may find it harder to speak. Their communication style may be very direct. Directness is appreciated in return, to avoid ambiguity in the information you are relaying to the person. If they are unable to speak or are struggling to speak easily, then a written/text app conversation might be preferred. Some autistic people use communication devices that are their spoken voice which reads out written text. They may also struggle to retain information, so make sure you can leave the information with them in multiple other ways to access: written, video, drawn, audio – make sure the information is as clear as possible. Above all else though, find out from the person themselves what they need from you for effective support and communication. Each autistic parent you meet will have different needs to the one you met before! Also be aware that the parent you are supporting may have done much reading and research and information-seeking, and that their knowledge may well be higher than the average parent you support!

Q: Is there anything you would want them to know about how autism can affect the breastfeeding relationship?

A: Sensory experiences will likely be the biggest factor in the breastfeeding relationship: the sensations of breastfeeding itself, the physical body closeness of baby/child to parent, the crying or screaming of a hungry baby, the frustrated baby who is struggling to latch.

Be aware that an autistic person who is sensitive to sounds may find that crying and screaming leaves them close to feeling utterly overwhelmed themselves. Their capacity to take in direction or information is going to be severely diminished. Consider carrying a stash of silicone earplugs in your bag (you can get multipacks cheaply online!) and offering them to an overwhelmed parent while you support them to calm the baby!

Touch can be a big deal for autistic parents. Many breast-feeding parents relate to being 'touched out'. This can be an even greater issue for an autistic parent. Exploring layering of clothes, and being open to carefully monitored use of nipple shields, pillows and creative positioning, can all help a parent feel less overwhelmed about being in frequent close contact with their baby.

Q: If a parent is breastfeeding an autistic child (whether post-diagnosis or pre-official diagnosis), do you think that brings additional challenges for a parent who is struggling and wants to bring in boundaries?

A: Parenting an autistic child generally requires disregarding the mainstream parenting information and advice that's out in the great wide world by the bucket load! Taking notice of what causes the child distress, what helps calm them, the sights, sounds and textures they seek out or avoid: all of these things can be used to help set up boundaries and routines that support a happy breastfeeding relationship. Be aware that an autistic child will be sensitive to their environment and may react with extreme distress if they feel unsafe and insecure.

Building *trust* with the child is key so that if breastfeeding isn't an option at that time, they can still experience security and comfort. That if 'this' thing doesn't happen, this 'other' thing *will* happen and that is also safe.

Q: What would you say to a parent who feels 'guilty' that they want to end breastfeeding, when their child values it as a regulation strategy?

A: The wellbeing of the parent matters too! Be prepared for the process of ending breastfeeding to take time. The age of the child and their level of communication can determine if you can make the ending of breastfeeding an effort of teamwork. Where possible, involve them in the process: even as simple as a counting game of sucks or minutes that you can tailor to the situation, and comforting distractions for afterwards.

Again, trust is key – that things can still be predictable and safe without breastfeeding.

Q: Are there any resources you would recommend?

A: • A Facebook group for Autistic Breastfeeding, Chest-feeding and Bodyfeeding Parents: www.facebook.com/groups/2231484463586660/
- Autistic Parents UK: www.autisticparentsuk.org/
- Autism Inclusivity (an autistic-led Facebook group for autistic people to lead education for non-autistic parents and carers): www.facebook.com/groups/autisminclusivity/
- Autistics Worldwide (an autistic-led Facebook group for general education for non-autistic people): www.facebook.com/groups/autisticsworldwide/

The best resources will come from those who are autistic parents themselves! An autistic parent may not even know they themselves are autistic if you are there to support a parent with an autistic child!

(Harper 2023)

How can we support a mother who is breastfeeding a child who is medically complex, when breastfeeding might be coming to an end? In her book *Breastfeeding the Brave*, Lyndsey Hookway shares some useful insights. In some cases, breastfeeding may be ending because of a child's medical issues, and managing a complex feeding situation alongside medical care is too challenging, and breastfeeding may be coming to an end reluctantly. It may be too much of a struggle to maintain milk supply while caring for other children and a child who is not well. Hookway reminds us:

> Humans are capable of holding two or more complex and sometimes slightly contradictory emotions at the same time. They can be relieved that the round-the-clock expressing for a child who is not capable of orally feeding is over, and also sad that their child will never directly breastfeed. (Hookway 2022, p.257)

Sometimes breastfeeding ends because a mother wants to stop. Hookway describes how some mothers agonize over whether it is 'fair' to deny their child breastmilk or the nurturing of breastfeeding: 'Feeling like breastfeeding will be the difference between health and illness, or life and death, can be an enormously overwhelming responsibility that leaves mothers unable to make a balanced and informed decision' (2022, p.258). Hookway suggests we frame the question differently: 'How long would they have to breastfeed for until they feel fully guilt-free about stopping? Is that length of time sensible or achievable?' (p.258).

In her book, Hookway goes into more detail about potentially considering some compromise options. Short of stopping completely, there are some scenarios which can mean a child receives some breastmilk, and smaller quantities will mean comparable concentrations of some immune factors as concentration increases. Essentially though, if a child has complex needs, there is a parent in the equation who needs to be protected. Parents need support to consider what will fill the gaps left behind when breastfeeding goes: new forms of nutrition and new forms of comfort and co-regulation. All parents need inner reserves to cope with caring for young children, even more so when there are additional challenges, and continuing to breastfeed beyond the point they want to brings risks. Breastfeeding will end for everyone eventually. The end may never be entirely 'guilt-free', but we can do our best to bring some perspective to the decision.

Chapter 12

Conclusion

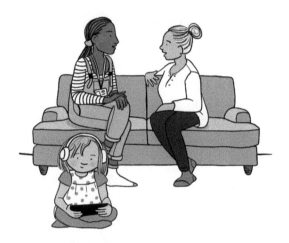

The Covid-19 pandemic transformed the way many breastfeeding supporters approached working with families, and weaning support has particularly benefitted from these new approaches. Online consultations using tools like Zoom mean that clients can come from a wide geographical range. A practitioner restricted to a small locality is unlikely to meet a large number of parents wishing to wean older children at any one time. Online meetings mean that sessions can be recorded. This can be valuable for a parent who may be describing some deep emotions and having some realizations for the first time that they may want to revisit or share with a partner. I have found it particularly successful to combine an initial consultation with ongoing WhatsApp support. In certain areas, there may be different considerations about security and privacy issues, but it is possible to find ways to communicate flexibly that suit both you and the families you support, and your professional requirements. Ongoing 'little and often' support can mean the breastfeeding supporter is a friendly ear in moments when parents are struggling to protect themselves, losing sight of their goals in the face of external pressure and finding it hard to know who else to talk to. An interaction may simply be:

'Last night he did wake, but he was happy to get back to sleep with a cuddle. It only took a few moments. I feel like we're turning a corner.'

'That sounds really positive. How are you feeling about tonight?'

'I'm thinking that we are ready for [my partner] to do some settling at night now. We've all been talking about it.'

'Those daytime conversations and preparation sound valuable. Good luck!'

Online options also make it easier for a peer group to form. I have organized several weaning peer-support groups that usually run for six to ten weeks, depending on the needs of the group. We meet weekly, again accompanied by a WhatsApp chat, which I tiptoe away from once the group has finished. Groups might centre around a particular age group or experience: for example, a group for pregnant parents looking to put in boundaries and explore what tandem feeding might look like. In this group, the majority did not choose to wean, but a peer group gave them a safe space to explore their options and be heard. Any weaning support must allow parents to change their minds. It might be helpful to term a group as 'weaning and exploring boundaries', rather than imply (once someone signs on the dotted line) that they are expected to stop breastfeeding within a certain time frame.

I also found during the pandemic that being outside and meeting parents for a walk was a valuable way to reflect on a weaning decision. Talking 'side-by-side' can mean more emotional sharing than talking 'face-to-face'. While the face-to-face conversation has the benefits of eye contact and a greater ability to read body language, talking side-by-side (particularly in a natural environment) can be freeing and allow parents to take time to be more reflective and pause naturally in conversation. On a practical level, walking can also happen with a toddler who is napping in a pushchair. Ideally, these conversations do not happen within earshot of a nursling. A parent needs to be able to speak openly and honestly and explore their options in a way that might leave a nursling feeling unsafe. I have occasionally had video calls where an older child was present. Screen times, headphones and code words made it possible to still have a valuable conversation.

If you are responsible for organizing local breastfeeding support services for a health service or volunteer organization, make space for conversations about the ending of breastfeeding. Mention it on your resources and in your groups. There are very few in the breastfeeding support world who don't understand that the heart of our work is about supporting families to reach their feeding goals. We have conversations about combination feeding and introducing formula on a return to work. We write in our Instagram profiles that we help parents to reach their goals. Our work must include supporting the stopping of breastfeeding. For many families, this will be the time they need us most. It may be the first time that they reach out to an infant feeding professional or volunteer after having an easy start to their breastfeeding journey. If we get this right, and we can support families at every stage of their journey, we have something to be proud of. We may be enabling parents to continue to offer breastmilk longer than they were expecting because they can now put boundaries in place and care for themselves.

Weaning support means enabling a parent to consider their needs as part of the breastfeeding experience, and the consequences of that can be far-reaching. If we don't support the transition from breastfeeding, different choices may be made the next time. I often speak to mothers who are struggling with the end of breastfeeding who declare that next time they won't even start co-sleeping or they will aim to break the feed-to-sleep association in infancy. This is what happens when support to end breastfeeding is lacking. Mothers are considering resisting the biological norm (and listening to some loud cultural voices which may not sit comfortably alongside breastfeeding) because the weaning process is challenging and isolating. Even if this ends up not happening, because the baby has other ideas, her next breastfeeding experience may be coloured by the fear that she is doing something 'wrong' and that the toughest bit is yet to come.

It is a woman's right to choose when she ends breastfeeding, and she is entitled to support to make that happen. We are certainly offering care that means mental health is protected, relationships are protected and families can lovingly move forward into the next stage of their parenting experience. Breastfeeding support is also the support not to breastfeed.

References

Aldort, N. (2005) *Raising Our Children, Raising Ourselves*. Bothell, WA: Book Publishers Network.

Australian Breastfeeding Association (2022) *Breastfeeding Rates in Australia*. Melbourne: Australian Breastfeeding Association. Accessed on 30/03/2023 at: www.breastfeeding.asn.au/resources/breastfeeding-rates-australia

Banks, S. (2022) *Why Formula Feeding Matters*. London: Pinter & Martin.

Bonyata, K. (2018) *Breastfeeding and Fertility*. Kellymom. Accessed on 30/03/2023 at: https://kellymom.com/ages/older-infant/fertility

Bonyata, K. (2022) *Do Babies Under Twelve Months Self-wean?* Kellymom. Accessed on 25/01/2023 at: https://kellymom.com/ages/older-infant/babyselfwean

Bonyata, K. (2023a) *Too Much Milk: Sage and Other Herbs for Decreasing Milk Supply*. Kellymom. Accessed on 20/02/2023 at: https://kellymom.com/bf/can-i-breastfeed/herbs/herbs-oversupply

Bonyata, K. (2023b) *How Much Expressed Milk Will My Baby Need?* Kellymom. Accessed on 15/01/2023 at: https://kellymom.com/bf/pumpingmoms/pumping/milkcalc/

Borra, C., Iacovou, M. and Sevilla, A. (2014) 'New evidence on breastfeeding and postpartum depression: the importance of understanding women's intentions.' *Maternal and Child Health Journal 19*, 897–907. doi: org/10.1007/s10995-014-1591-z

Borresen, K. (2022) *How to Wean from Breastfeeding, According to Lactation Experts*. London: Huffington Post. Accessed on 27/10/2022 at: https://www.huffingtonpost.co.uk/entry/tips-weaning-breastfeeding-lactation-experts_l_63338b6ae4b028164523b6aa

Breastfeed LA (2019, November 17) Facebook. Accessed on 30.3.2023 at: https://www.facebook.com/BreastfeedLA/photos/in-a-zoo-in-ohio-a-female-gorilla-was-born-and-raised-in-captivity-got-pregnant-/2556713934382316

Breastfeeding for Doctors (2022) *Position Statement on the Shared Caregiving of the Breastfed Child*. London: Breastfeeding for Doctors. Accessed on 16/01/2022 at: https://breastfeedingfordoctors.com/wp-content/uploads/2022/06/BFD-Shared-Caregiving-Breastfed-Child-Statement.pdf

The Breastfeeding Network (2019) *Drugs in Breastmilk: Is It Safe?* Paisley: Breastfeeding Network. Accessed on 18/04/2023 at: www.breastfeedingnetwork.org.uk/detailed-information/drugs-in-breastmilk

The Breastfeeding Network (2022) *Antidepressants and Breastfeeding*. Paisley: The Breastfeeding Network. Accessed on 18/04/2023 at: www.breastfeedingnetwork.org.uk/antidepressants

Brown, A. (2019) *Why Breastfeeding Grief and Trauma Matter*. London: Pinter & Martin.

Brown, A. (2021) *Let's Talk about Feeding Your Baby*. London: Pinter & Martin.

Brown, A. (2022) *The Compassion Code: Power, Perseverance and Passion in Lactation Support*. London: TR Books.

Brown, A. and Harries, V. (2015) 'Infant sleep and night feeding patterns during later infancy: association with breastfeeding frequency, daytime complementary food intake, and infant weight.' *Breastfeeding Medicine* 10, 5, 246–252. doi: org/10.1089/bfm.2014.0153

Centers for Disease Control and Prevention (2022a) *Breastfeeding Report Card*. Washington DC: US Department of Health and Human Services. Accessed on 17/12/2022 at: www.cdc.gov/breastfeeding/data/reportcard.htm

Centers for Disease Control and Prevention (2022b) *Cow's Milk and Milk Alternatives*. Washington DC: US Department of Health and Human Services. Accessed on 30/03/2023 at: www.cdc.gov/nutrition/InfantandToddlerNutrition/foods-and-drinks/cows-milk-and-milk-alternatives.html

Clarke, S. (2023a) Email with Emma Pickett, 9 March.

Clarke, S. (2023b) *21 Days of Play*. Shelley Clarke. Accessed on 18/04/2023 at: https://shelleyclarke.newzenler.com/courses/21-days-of-play

Cohen, L. (2012) *Playful Parenting*. New York: Ballantine Books.

Cox, J. (2021) *Paternity Leave: The Hidden Barriers Keeping Men at Work*. London: BBC Worklife. Accessed on 19/12/2022 at: https://www.bbc.com/worklife/article/20210712-paternity-leave-the-hidden-barriers-keeping-men-at-work

De Visscher, M. (2020) *Bye-Bye Mommy's Milk*. Istanbul: Kütüphaneler ve Yayımlar Genel Müdürlüğü.

Dewey, K.G. (2001) 'Nutrition, growth, and complementary feeding of the breast-fed infant.' *Pediatric Clinics of North America* 48, 1, 87–104. doi: 10.1016/s0031-3955(05)70287-x

Dillemuth, J. (2017) *Loving Comfort: A Toddler Weaning Story*. Santa Barbara, CA: Julie Dillemuth.

Dowling, S. (2018) '"Betwixt and Between": Women's Experiences of Breastfeeding Long Term,' in S. Dowling, D. Pontin, and K. Boyer (eds) *Social Experiences of Breastfeeding: Building Bridges between Research, Policy and Practice*. Bristol: Policy Press Scholarship, pp.55–70. doi.org/10.1332/policypress/9781447338499.003.0005

Elder, J. (2020) *My Milk Will Go, Our Love Will Grow*. USA: Heart Words Press.

First Steps Nutrition Trust (2014, updated 2020) *Eating Well: Vegan Infants and Under-5s*. London: First Steps Nutrition Trust. Accessed on 29/03/2023 at: https://static1.squarespace.com/static/59f75004f09ca48694070f3b/t/5e56fa31f3d-6f227ed61362c/1582758484838/Eating_well_Vegans-Feb_2020_forweb.pdff

First Steps Nutrition Trust (2015, reprinted 2020) *Eating Well: The First Year*. London: First Steps Nutrition Trust. Accessed on 29/03/2023 at: www.firststepsnutrition.org/eating-well-infants-new-mums

First Steps Nutrition Trust (2020) *Infant Formula: An Overview*. London: First Steps Nutrition Trust. Accessed on 06/02/2023 at: https://infantmilkinfo.org/wp-content/uploads/2020/03/Infant-formula_overview_final.pdf

First Steps Nutrition Trust (2021a) *Follow-on Formula*. London: First Steps Nutrition Trust. https://infantmilkinfo.org/wp-content/uploads/2021/10/Follow_on-Formula_October2021.pdf

First Steps Nutrition Trust (2021b) *Infant Milks: A Simple Guide to Infant Formula, Follow-on Formula and Other Infant Milks*. London: First Steps Nutrition Trust. Accessed on 6/02/2023 at: www.firststepsnutrition.org/parents-carers

First Steps Nutrition Trust (2022a) *Costs of Infant Formula, Follow-on Formula and Milks Marketed as Foods for Special Medical Purposes Available Over the Counter in the UK*. London: First Steps Nutrition Trust. https://infantmilkinfo.org/costs/

First Steps Nutrition Trust (2022b) *The Bacterial Contamination of Powdered Infant Formula*. London: First Steps Nutrition Trust. www.firststepsnutrition.org/making-infant-milk-safely

Flower, H. (2018) *Getting Pregnant While Breastfeeding*. Kellymom. Accessed on 30/03/2023 at: https://kellymom.com/ages/older-infant/ttc-while-bf

Flower, H. (2019) *Adventures in Tandem Nursing: Breastfeeding during Pregnancy and Beyond*. Raleigh, NC: La Leche League International.

Food Safety Authority of Ireland (2021) *Using Expressed Breastmilk or Infant Formula Safely*. Dublin: Food Safety Authority of Ireland. Accessed on 25/01/2023 at: www.fsai.ie/faq/bottle_feeding_safely.html

Glaser, E. (2022) *Motherhood: Feminism's Unfinished Business*. London: Fourth Estate.

Global Health Media (2016) *Cup Feeding* [Video]. Global Health Media. Accessed on 30/03/2023 at: https://globalhealthmedia.org/videos/cup-feeding

Gordon, J. (2020) 'Sleep, Changing Patterns in the Family Bed.' *Jay Gordon, MD, FAAP*. Accessed on 24/01/2023 at: www.drjaygordon.com/blog-detail/sleep-changing-patterns-in-the-family-bed

Grant, A. (2022) *How Midwifery Staff Can Support Autistic Women with Breastfeeding: Recommendations from Autistic People*. Maternity & Midwifery Forum. Accessed on 06/02/23 at: www.maternityandmidwifery.co.uk/how-midwifery-staff-can-support-autistic-women-with-breastfeeding

Grant, A., Jones, S., Sibson, V., Ellis, R. *et al.* (2023) 'The safety of at home powdered infant formula preparation: A community science project.' *Maternal & Child Nutrition*, e13567. https://doi.org/10.1111/mcn.13567

Grant, A. and Williams, K. (2022) *Autistic Mothers' Experiences of Breast- and Formula-feeding Babies: What Does the Evidence Say?* Autistic UK. Accessed on 06/02/2023 at: www.autisticuk.org/post/autistic-mothers-experiences-of-breast-and-formula-feeding-babies-what-does-the-evidence-s

Grueger, B., Canadian Paediatric Society and Community Paediatrics Committee (2013) 'Weaning from the breast.' *Paediatrics & Child Health* 18, 4, p.210. doi.org/10.1093/pch/18.4.210

Hand in Hand Parenting (2023) Accessed on 18/04/2023 at: https://www.handinhand-parenting.org/

Hardwicke, E. (2021) *A Big Change for Seb*. Halifax, West Yorkshire: Fi and Books.

Harper, B. (2023) Email with Emma Pickett, 10 February.

Harris, K., Murphy, K.E., Horn, D., MacGilivray, J. *et al.* (2020) 'Safety of cabergoline for postpartum lactation inhibition or suppression: a systematic review.' *Journal of Obstetrics and Gynaecology Canada* 42, 3, 308–315.e20. doi.org/10.1016/j.jogc.2019.03.014

Havener, K. (2013) *Nursies When the Sun Shines*. Santa Clarita, CA: Elea Press.

Health and Social Care Information Centre (2012) *Infant Feeding Survey 2010*. Leeds: NHS Digital. https://files.digital.nhs.uk/publicationimport/pub08xxx/pub08694/infant-feeding-survey-2010-consolidated-report.pdf

Hookway, L. (2018) *Holistic Sleep Coaching: Gentle Alternatives to Sleep Training for Health and Childcare Professionals*. Amarillo, TX: Praeclarus Press.

Hookway, L. (2021) *Still Awake: Responsive Sleep Tools for Toddlers to Tweens*. London: Pinter & Martin.

Hookway, L. (2022) *Breastfeeding the Brave*. London: Thought Rebellion.

Jindal, S., Gao, D., Bell, P., Albrektsen, G. *et al.* (2014) 'Postpartum breast involution reveals regression of secretory lobules mediated by tissue-remodeling.' *Breast Cancer Research 16*, R31. doi.org/10.1186/bcr3633

Johnson, H.M., Eglash, A., Mitchell, K.B., Leeper, K. *et al.* (2020) 'ABM Clinical Protocol #32: Management of hyperlactation.' *Breastfeeding Medicine 15*, 3, 129–134. doi.org/10.1089/bfm.2019.29141.hmj

Jones, W. (2018) *Breastfeeding and Medication*. Abingdon: Routledge.

Kernerman, E. (2011) *Solving Breast Refusal and Inability to Latch*. York, ON: International Breastfeeding Centre. Accessed on 20/12/2022 at: https://ibconline.ca/wp-content/uploads/2016/06/Not-Yet-Latching-Baby-Notes.pdf

Kippley, S. and Kippley, J. (1972) 'The relation between breastfeeding and amenorrhea: report of a survey.' *Journal of Obstetric, Gynecologic, and Neonatal Nursing 1*, 4, 15–21. doi: org/10.1111/j.1552-6909.1972.tb00558.x

La Leche League International (2020) *Fertility*. Raleigh, NC: La Leche League International. www.llli.org/breastfeeding-info/fertility

La Leche League International (2021) *Menstruation*. Raleigh, NC: La Leche League International. Accessed on 30/03/2023 at: www.llli.org/breastfeeding-info/menstruation

La Leche League International (2022) *Cancer: Diagnostic Tests, Therapeutic Procedures and Treatment While Breastfeeding*. Raleigh, NC: La Leche League International. Accessed on 16/01/2023 at: https://www.llli.org/breastfeeding-info/cancer-diagnostic-tests-therapeutic-procedures-and-treatment-while-breastfeeding

Leon-Joyce, A. (2022) Conversation with Emma Pickett, 10 November.

Lorick, G. (2009) 'Life Is Full of Weanings.' *Conservative Granola Mommies*, 2 March. Accessed on 27/01/2023 at: https://conservativegranolamommies.blogspot.com/2009/03/life-is-full-of-weanings.html

McKenna, J.J. and Gettler, L.T. (2016) 'There is no such thing as infant sleep, there is no such thing as breastfeeding, there is only breastsleeping.' *Acta Paediatrica 105*, 17–21. doi.org/10.1111/apa.13161

Mitchell, K.B., Johnson, H.M., Rodríguez, J.M., Eglash, A. *et al.* (2022) 'Academy of Breastfeeding Medicine Clinical Protocol #36: the mastitis spectrum, revised 2022.' *Breastfeeding Medicine 17*, 5, 360–376. doi: 10.1089/bfm.2022.29207.kbm

Mitchell, L. (2013) *Sally Weans from Night Nursing*. USA: Create Space Independent Publishing Platform.

Mohrbacher, N. (2020) *Breastfeeding Answers: A Guide for Helping Families*. Arlington Heights, IL: Nancy Mohrbacher Solutions.

Mooney, R. (2021) Conversation with Emma Pickett, 28 April.

NHS (2019) *Formula Milk: Common Questions*. Accessed on 30/03/2023 at: NHS. www.nhs.uk/conditions/baby/breastfeeding-and-bottle-feeding/bottle-feeding/formula-milk-questions/

NHS Better Health Start for Life (2023) *What to Feed Your Baby*. London: NHS Public Health England. Accessed on 30/03/2023 at: www.nhs.uk/start4life/weaning/what-to-feed-your-baby/7-9-months

NSPCC (2012) *Tips and Advice to Help Keep Your Kids Safe*. London: National Society for the Prevention of Cruelty to Children. Accessed on 20/01/2023 at: www.nspcc.org.uk/keeping-children-safe/support-for-parents/pants-underwear-rule

Ockwell-Smith, S. (2013) *ToddlerCalm: A Guide for Calmer Toddlers and Happier Parents*. London: Piatkus.

Osei-Barrett, N. and Riley, C. (2021) *Boobies Go Bye-Bye: A Weaning Story*. Arizona: Matriarch Press.

Palou, M., Picó, C. and Palou, A. (2018) 'Leptin as a breast milk component for the prevention of obesity.' *Nutrition Reviews* 76, 12, 875–892. doi.org/10.1093/nutrit/nuy046

Pearson-Glaze, P. (2022) *Tips to Bottle Feed a Breastfed Baby*. UK: Breastfeeding.support. Accessed on 16/12/2022 at: https://breastfeeding.support/tips-to-bottle-feed-a-breastfed-baby

Perry, P. (2020) *The Book You Wish Your Parents Had Read (and Your Children Will Be Glad That You Did)*. London: Penguin Life.

Perry, P. (2022) 'I'm Now Sober, but Feel Guilty about a Friend I've Left Behind.' *The Guardian*, 13 November. www.theguardian.com/lifeandstyle/2022/nov/13/ask-philippa-perry-i-am-now-sober-but-feel-guilty-about-a-friend-i-left-behind

Pickett, E. (2014) *Weaning Toddler Bob and Pre-schooler Billie: How Do You Stop Breastfeeding an Older Child?* Accessed on 30/03/2023 at: www.emmapickettbreastfeedingsupport.com/twitter-and-blog/weaning-toddler-bob-and-pre-schooler-billie-how-do-you-stop-breastfeeding-an-older-child

Pickett, E. (2022) *Supporting Breastfeeding Past the First Six Months and Beyond: A Guide for Professionals and Parents*. London: Jessica Kingsley Publishers.

Pisacane, A., Continisio, P. and the Italian Work Group on Breastfeeding (2004) 'Breastfeeding and perceived changes in the appearance of the breasts: a retrospective study.' *Acta Paediatrica* 93, 10, 1346–1348. https://doi.org/10.1080/08035250410033880

Pride, C. (2011) *Vitamin B6 Vasospasm*. Lubbock, TX: InfantRisk Center, Texas Tech University Health Sciences Center. Accessed on 30/03/2023 at: www.infantrisk.com/forum/forum/medications-and-breastfeeding-mothers/vitamins/358-vitamin-b6-vasospasm

Public Health Scotland (2021) *Infant Feeding Statistics*. Glasgow: Public Health Scotland. Accessed on 30/03/2023 at: https://publichealthscotland.scot/publications/infant-feeding-statistics/infant-feeding-statistics-financial-year-2020-to-2021

Ransom, N. (2023) 'I've Stopped Saying I "Have Autism" – For Me, Being Autistic Is Brilliant, Not a Burden.' *The Guardian*, 6 February. Accessed on 06/02/2023 at: www.theguardian.com/commentisfree/2023/feb/06/autism-autistic-positive-neurodiversity

Regan, L. (2018) *What Are Miscarriage and Preterm Labor Experts Saying?* Kellymom. https://kellymom.com/tandem-faq/02miscarriage

Reid, Y. (2021) *Booby Moon: A Weaning Book for Toddlers*. Wellington: New Zealand ISBN Agency.

Reid, Y. (2022) *Booby Moon with Two: A Storybook for Gently Weaning Tandem-fed Toddlers*. Wellington: New Zealand ISBN Agency.

Reilly, J. (2022) Email with Emma Pickett, 3 November.

Rice, R. (2017) *Bye-Bye Nah-Nahs*. San Diego, CA: Easy Tiger Books.

Rose, M. and Stone, L. (2019, 17 November) 'Food and control' (No. 28) [Podcast episode]. *The Aware Parenting Podcast*. https://podcasts.apple.com/gb/podcast/episode-28-food-and-control/id1455772681?i=1000457016739

Saleem, J. (2014) *Milkies in the Morning*. USA: Jennifer Saleem Books.

Saunt, R. (2023) 'Orangutan Finally Learned How To Nurse Her Baby Thanks to Zookeeper.' *Daily Mail*, 31 March. www.dailymail.co.uk/femail/article-11925695/amp/Orangutan-finally-learned-nurse-new-baby-thanks-breastfeeding-zookeeper.html

Schummers, L., Hutcheon, J.A., Hernandez-Diaz, S., Williams, P.L. *et al.* (2018) 'Association of short interpregnancy interval with pregnancy outcomes according to maternal age.' *Journal of the American Medical Association Internal Medicine* 178, 12, 1661–1670. doi:10.1001/jamainternmed.2018.4696

Scottish Government (2017) *Scottish Maternal and Infant Nutrition Survey 2017.* Edinburgh: Scottish Government. Accessed on 30/03/2023 at: www.gov.scot/binaries/content/documents/govscot/publications/statistics/2018/02/scottish-maternal-infant-nutrition-survey-2017/documents/00531610-pdf/00531610-pdf/govscot:document/00531610.pdf

Solter, A.J. (1998) *Tears and Tantrums: What To Do When Babies and Children Cry.* Goleta, CA: Shining Star Press.

Solter, A. (2022) *What Is Aware Parenting?* Aware Parenting Institute. http://aware-parenting.com

Susan, M. (2018) *A Time To Wean.* USA: Corolishine Books.

UNICEF (2018) 'On Mother's Day, UNICEF calls for the narrowing of 'breastfeeding gaps' between rich and poor worldwide' [Media release] 10 May. Accessed on 17/12/2022 at: www.unicef.org/press-releases/mothers-day-unicef-calls-narrowing-breastfeeding-gaps-between-rich-and-poor

UNICEF UK Baby Friendly Initiative (2018) *Breastfeeding: A Mother's Gift for Every Child.* London: UNICEF UK. Accessed on 17/12/2022 at: www.unicef.org.uk/babyfriendly/breastfeeding-mothers-gift-every-child

UNICEF UK Baby Friendly Initiative (2019) *Responsive Bottle Feeding.* London: UNICEF UK. Accessed on 24/01/2023 at: www.unicef.org.uk/babyfriendly/wp-content/uploads/sites/2/2019/04/Infant-formula-and-responsive-bottle-feeding.pdf

UNICEF UK Baby Friendly Initiative (2023a) *About the Baby Friendly Initiative.* London: UNICEF UK. Accessed on 30/03/2023 at: www.unicef.org.uk/babyfriendly/about

UNICEF UK Baby Friendly Initiative (2023b) *Overweight and Obesity Infant Health Research.* London: UNICEF UK. Accessed on 21/02/2023 at: www.unicef.org.uk/babyfriendly/news-and-research/baby-friendly-research/infant-health-research/infant-health-research-obesity

University Hospitals of Leicester (2021) *Lactation Suppression.* Leicester: University Hospitals of Leicester NHS Trust. Accessed on 28/01/2023 at: https://secure.library.leicestershospitals.nhs.uk/PAGL/SharedDocuments/LactationSuppressionFollowingBereavementUHLObstetricGuideline.pdf

Wambach, K. and Riordan, J. (2016) *Breastfeeding and Human Lactation.* Fifth edition. Burlington, MA: Jones and Barlett Learning.

Weeks, M. (2022) *Goodbye Mummy's Milk.* London: Mariapaola Weeks.

Weschler, T. (2016) *Taking Charge of Your Fertility.* Revised edition. London: Vermillion, Ebury.

Wolfarth, J. (2023) *Milk: An Intimate History of Breastfeeding.* London: Weidenfeld and Nicolson.

Wong, B.B., Koh, S. and Gail, D. (2012) 'The effectiveness of cabbage leaf application (treatment) on pain and hardness in breast engorgement and its effect on the duration of breastfeeding.' *JBI Library of Systematic Reviews* 10, 20, 1185–1213. doi: 10.11124/jbisrir-2012-58

Wong, B.B., Chan, Y.H., Leow, M., Lu, Y. *et al.* (2017) 'Application of cabbage leaves compared to gel packs for mothers with breast engorgement: randomised controlled trial.' *International Journal of Nursing Studies* 76, 92–99. doi.org/10.1016/j.ijnurstu.2017.08.014

Wood, B. and Tenner, J. (2022, October 26) 'How do I be my own anchor in my perfect storm?' (No. 383) [Podcast episode]. *Nourishing the Mother.* https://podcasts.apple.com/gb/podcast/nourishing-the-mother/id1013746031?i=1000583902440

Woodstein, B.J. (2022) Conversation with Emma Pickett, 29 November.

World Economic Forum (2022) *COVID-19 Lockdowns Saw Couples Share Housework and Childcare More Evenly – But Not for Long.* Geneva: World Economic Forum. Accessed on 19/12/2022 at www.weforum.org/agenda/2022/01/gender-equality-domestic-labor-housework-family-men-women-lockdown

Zia, S. (2022) 'For Autistic Mothers, Breastfeeding is Complicated.' *New York Times,* 4 October. Accessed on 10/10/2022 at: www.nytimes.com/2022/10/04/health/formula-shortage-autism-breastfeeding.html

Further Resources

Weaning picture books

De Visscher, M. (2020) *Bye-Bye Mommy's Milk*. Istanbul: Kütüphaneler ve Yayımlar Genel Müdürlüğü.

Dillemuth, J. (2017) *Loving Comfort: A Toddler Weaning Story*. Santa Barbara, CA: Julie Dillemuth.

'Don't offer, Don't refuse': www.emmapickettbreastfeedingsupport.com/twitter-and-blog/dont-offer-dont-refuse

Elder, J. (2020) *My Milk Will Go, Our Love Will Grow*. USA: Heart Words Press.

Hardwicke, E. (2021) *A Big Change for Seb*. Halifax: Fi and Books.com

Havener, K. (2013) *Nursies When the Sun Shines*. Santa Clarita, CA: Elea Press.

Mitchell, L. (2013) *Sally Weans from Night Nursing*. USA: Create Space Independent Publishing Platform.

Osei-Barrett, N. and Riley, C. (2021) *Boobies Go Bye-Bye: A Weaning Story*. Arizona, USA: Matriarch Press.

Reid, Y. (2021) *Booby Moon: A Weaning Book for Toddlers*. Wellington: New Zealand ISBN Agency.

Reid, Y. (2022) *Booby Moon with Two: A Storybook for Gently Weaning Tandem-fed Toddlers*. Wellington: New Zealand ISBN Agency.

Rice, R. (2017) *Bye-Bye Nah-Nahs*. San Diego, CA: Easy Tiger Books.

Saleem, J. (2014) *Milkies in the Morning*. USA: Jennifer Saleem Books.

Saunt, R. (2023) 'Orangutan Finally Learned How To Nurse Her Baby Thanks to Zoo-keeper.' *Daily Mail*, 31 March. www.dailymail.co.uk/femail/article-11925695/amp/Orangutan-finally-learned-nurse-new-baby-thanks-breastfeeding-zookeeper.html

Susan, M. (2018) *A Time To Wean*. USA: Corolishine Books.

Weeks, M. (2022) *Goodbye Mummy's Milk*. London: Mariapaola Weeks.

Further articles by Emma

Toddler Breastfeeding in Lockdown (setting boundaries): https://www.emmapickettbreastfeedingsupport.com/twitter-and-blog/category/toddler-breastfeeding-in-lockdown

Toddler Twiddling: https://thenaturalparentmagazine.com/toddler-twiddling/

Weaning Toddler Bob and pre-schooler Billie: www.emmapickettbreastfeedingsupport.com/twitter-and-blog/category/weaning-toddler-bob-and-preschooler-billie-howdo-you-stop-breastfeeding-an-older-child

Subject Index

Author Index